Shortness of Breath

A Guide to Better Living and Breathing

Shortness of Breath

A Guide to Better Living and Breathing

Andrew L. Ries, MD, MPH

Patricia J. Bullock, RRT, RCP

Catherine A. Larsen, MPH

Trina M. Limberg, BS, RRT, RCP

Roseann Myers, RN, BSN

Toni Pfister, MS

Dawn E. Sassi-Dambron, RN, BSN

Jamie B. Sheldon, PT

Pulmonary Rehabilitation Program
Division of Pulmonary and Critical Care Medicine
University of California, San Diego
School of Medicine
San Diego, California

SIXTH EDITION

Illustrations by Steve Pileggi

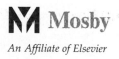

An Affiliate of Elsevier

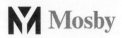

An Affiliate of Elsevier

ACQUISITIONS EDITOR Karen Fabiano
DEVELOPMENTAL EDITOR Mindy Copeland
PROJECT MANAGER Karen Edwards
DESIGNER Stephanie Foley
COVER ART The Stock Market

SIXTH EDITION

NOTICE

Pharmacology in an ever-changing field. Standard safety precautions must be followed, but as new research and clinical experience broaden our knowledge, changes in treatment and drug therapy become necessary or appropriate. Readers are advised to check the product information currently provided by the manufacturer of each drug to be administered to verify the recommended dose, the method and duration of administration, and the contraindications. It is the responsibility of the treating physician, relying on experience and knowledge of the patient, to determine dosages and the best treatment for the patient. Neither the publisher nor the authors assume any responsibility for any injury and/or damage to persons or property.

Permissions may be sought directly from Elsevier's Health Sciences Rights Department in Philadelphia, PA, USA: phone: (+1) 215 239 3804, fax: (+1) 215 239 3805, e-mail: healthpermissions@elsevier.com. You may also complete your request on-line via the Elsevier homepage (http://www.elsevier.com), by selecting 'Customer Support' and then 'Obtaining Permissions'.

Mosby, Inc.
An Affiliate of Elsevier
11830 Westline Industrial Drive
St. Louis, Missouri 63146

Printed in the United States of America

Library of Congress Cataloging-in-Publication Data

Shortness of breath: a guide to better living and breathing / Andrew L. Ries . . . [et al.].—6th ed.
    p. cm.
    ISBN-13: 978-0-323-01064-1   ISBN-10: 0-323-01064-4 (soft cover)
        1. Lungs—Diseases, Obstructive—Popular works. I. Ries, Andrew L.
    RC776.O3 S53 2000
    616.2'4—dc21

                                                                00-040197

ISBN-13: 978-0-323-01064-1
ISBN-10: 0-323-01064-4

06 07 08 09 GW/MV 9 8 7 6 5

To

Kenneth M. Moser, MD

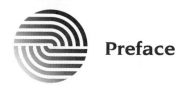

Preface

Any book with multiple authors of different backgrounds must have an interesting story behind it, and this one does. The story began more than 30 years ago, when Dr. Kenneth M. Moser, the inspiration and guiding light for this book, established one of the first respiratory intensive care units in the United States. Trying to save the lives of patients who had developed severe, life-threatening breathing problems was a rewarding and exciting venture. Yet it was soon recognized that many admissions to this unit and to the hospital could have been avoided if the patient had, long before, understood better the causes of breathing problems and how to deal with them. Dr. Moser and the other dedicated staff members working with him at the time decided that educating patients was a vital and missing link in the health care system. At the time, persons with breathing problems were, almost exclusively, *passive observers* of their own health care. Dr. Moser and his colleagues became convinced that with proper education, people could and should become *active participants* in their own health care.

But how could laypeople acquire such education? Certainly not through medical textbooks, which were too technical and detailed. Nor through the standard media, which dealt only sporadically with breathing problems and rarely presented practical or scientifically sound information. Nor from most health books," which usually presented a point of view rather than a body of facts. And not from busy physicians or other health professionals who, however well-motivated, rarely had time to educate their patients. Furthermore, many persons with breathing problems did not know when or whether to enter the health care system and, therefore, often entered it at a late stage with advanced problems. Over the years the health care system has changed, but these issues remain. As more and more people have developed lung disease—a real "growth industry" in the twentieth century—patients' need for reliable and *readable* information has also grown.

From the beginning, we concluded that such an educational effort could be provided most effectively by a team of health professionals that included persons with a wide range of professional skills and knowledge: pulmonary physicians, pulmonary nursing specialists, respiratory therapists, chest physical therapists, exercise specialists, cardiopulmonary technologists, psychiatrists and psychologists, social workers, nutritionists, pharmacists, occupational therapists, hospital administrators, and others. This team would develop a program devoted to the education and training of patients with breathing problems—*and their families*—emphasizing the most common cause of this symptom, chronic obstructive pulmonary disease (COPD), but not neglecting patients with other forms of chronic lung disease.

In the beginning, such ideas and approaches were controversial. Some believed that an educated patient might be more of a threat than a help to the health care system; others believed that people would not be interested in such self-education. Still others thought that such an effort would intrude on doctor-patient relationships. Despite such reservations, the effort was undertaken.

The multidisciplinary team was developed and together designed a pulmonary rehabilitation program for people with shortness of breath and other breathing problems. The first patients came, learned, and benefited. The process was refined, changed, and repeated, and a gratifying dividend appeared. As the years and programs passed, many physicians and other health professionals visited our rehabilitation program to learn the elements and began similar efforts at their offices, clinics, and hospitals. Research studies conducted at the University of California San Diego and elsewhere have established the scientific basis of pulmonary rehabilitation and shown that patients really do benefit from this approach.

Our efforts were still reaching a relatively small audience, however, which was an increasing source of frustration. Our program was consistently "backlogged," so that we could reach only a modest percentage of the interested persons in our immediate geographic area. Many persons with lung disease did not have access to such programs, and extension of our program to other areas was not feasible. This book was a logical means for extending our educational efforts to the larger audience that we could never reach in person. That is the story behind the first edition of this book, which appeared in 1975.

With each succeeding edition, we have asked those who have used this manual to help us make it more valuable to them. We have listened closely to their suggestions this time as well. In addition, there have been medical advances in our understanding of the multiple lung diseases that can cause symptoms, as well as improvements in treatment. One among many such advances has been the expanded availability and feasibility of surgical operations, such as lung transplantation, for many patients with advanced breathing problems. It has been found that participation in a rehabilitation program is a key element in the preparation of such patients for surgery and in their postoperative recovery.

Thus over the years this book—like all aspects of medical care—has changed. One thing, however, has not changed; indeed it has become stronger and is still the theme of this book: our belief that persons with breathing problems can become active members of the treatment team, accepting (and enjoying) the fact that they can and must play a central role in their own care.

We hope that all of our colleagues in medicine will continue to find this book useful and that patients with breathing problems will learn from its pages how to live better and more functional lives.

Of course, in addition to the multiple authors of this edition, many others have contributed much, directly or indirectly, to this book. We owe special debts of gratitude to Steve Pileggi, who has provided the illustrations for this book and for our programs since the first edition and who has updated and added many for this edition. In particular, we would like to thank the former staff members of the UCSD Pulmonary Rehabilitation Program who over the years have contributed so much to the development of the program and who have been authors and contributors to previous editions of this book: Carol Archibald, RN; Deon Dunn, RN; Marion Modrak, RN; Patsy Hansen, RN; Alice Beamon, RT; Birgitta Ellis, PT; Donna Whelan, RT; Martin Davis, RT; and Lynn Johnson, RN. Among the psychiatrists and psychologists who have devoted themselves to the mental health of our patients (and ourselves) are Stephen Groban, MD; Alan Abrams, MD; and Sharon Grodner, Ph.D. Of the many allied health professionals who have provided so much of their knowledge, experience, and themselves, we would particularly like to thank dieticians Joyce Knott and Kelly Mosier, who have taught our patients and us so much about nutrition; pharmacists Richard Levy, Raffi Simonian, Ken Schell, Joanne Goralka, and Marcie Lepkowsky for straightening us all out about the proper use of medications; Jane Villareal, a social worker whose caring and understanding were exemplary; and a succession of pulmonary trainees and students at UCSD who have been our teachers as well as our students. Nancy Dimsdale contributed illustrations for previous editions. For the publication of this book, we owe much to Lela Prewitt, who has borne the administrative burdens. Finally, most of all, we owe thanks to our many patients who have continued to return to us far more than we have given to them.

There is one aspect of this sixth edition that is different from those that preceded it. This is the first edition completed without Kenneth M. Moser's guiding hand. Dr. Moser passed away in 1997. He not only was the inspiration for this book and the pulmonary rehabilitation program from which it was developed but also was the inspiration, mentor, and guiding light for all of us and for the many health professionals who contributed to the earlier editions. Dr. Moser was always a man who looked forward and who took great pride in "passing the torch" to future generations of physicians and other health professionals who trained and worked under his nurturing spirit. Carrying this book—and his work—forward is not only what Dr. Moser would want but also what he would expect. In that spirit, we dedicate this book to Dr. Moser and commit our efforts to improving the lives of those patients we have had the privilege to serve and those many others who may benefit from the accumulated wisdom set forth in these pages. As Dr. Moser himself would say, "God Bless!"

Andrew L. Ries, MD, MPH

Contents in Brief

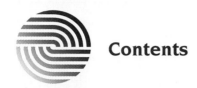 **Contents**

1

What Are Shortness of Breath and Other Breathing Problems All About?

Most of us take breathing for granted. Like the beating of the heart, breathing just happens automatically. When we exercise, we know our breathing quickens and deepens, just as our pulse rate increases. But, again, we don't have to think about these things. We decide what we want to do, and somehow the lungs (and heart) follow along.

The medical word for feeling short of breath is *dyspnea* (pronounced disp'-nee-ah). Dyspnea is a difficult symptom for people to deal with because it is a feeling, a sensation of breathing discomfort or air hunger. Only the patient knows that he or she is experiencing shortness of breath. The physician also can have difficulty evaluating dyspnea. It cannot be detected on physical examination. There is no specific test for it. Therefore, the patient must report dyspnea to the physician. In many ways, dyspnea is like pain—a symptom that only the patient feels and can describe. Pain and dyspnea are invisible to others.

Like pain, shortness of breath is experienced differently by different people. Some persons have a very high threshold for pain, some a very low one. It is the same with dyspnea. Some people who appear to others to be short of breath do not themselves feel dyspneic. Others feel quite short of breath when they appear to be breathing normally. Just why this is cannot be fully explained. There are probably multiple reasons.

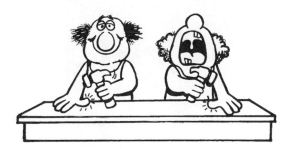

WHEN IS SHORTNESS OF BREATH ABNORMAL?

So shortness of breath is a tricky symptom. To compound the problem, everyone feels short of breath sometimes. Even the well-conditioned athlete with excellent lung and heart function experiences dyspnea. So how do you know when shortness of breath is abnormal? When is it a possible signal of disease? When should you have it checked out by a doctor? Here are some simple tests to apply:

1. Are you more short of breath doing certain things than other people your own age? It is obviously not abnormal when a 60-year-old man or woman feels short of breath while playing tennis with a 20-year-old son or daughter. It is not abnormal to feel short of breath if you lead a quite sedentary life and suddenly try to run a mile. But it is abnormal if you feel short of breath walking up an incline or up stairs when people of your own age (co-workers, friends, or spouse) do not. Comparison with peers is a key test.

2. Are you short of breath doing things that a few months or a year ago you could do easily without this feeling? Do you now avoid the stairs at work or at home because of shortness of breath? In asking these questions, you are comparing you with yourself. The questions should be answered honestly. Denying such changes won't make them go away.

3. Have you experienced a sudden change? Suddenly feeling short of breath at rest or with activity is almost always abnormal. A rapid change such as this merits prompt medical attention.

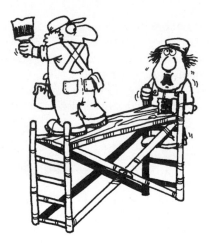

Asking these questions usually distinguishes normal from abnormal shortness of breath. Sometimes, though, a person either does not ask these questions or denies that the answers are "yes." Unconsciously, you may cut back on what you are doing to avoid shortness of breath. Or you may attribute the symptoms to just "getting older" or being out of shape. In such situations, other people may call the problem to your attention. They notice that you may be breathing hard during a walk at a pace that is leisurely for them.

Friends or spouses are often the first to notice such things. If others pose these questions to you, take them seriously rather than explaining them away (which is easy to do). You may have a high threshold for breathing discomfort, but if you are changing your behavior to avoid shortness of breath, others may be more aware of it than you are. Or maybe you are aware, but don't want to admit it as long as you believe that no one else notices.

CHECK IT OUT

However shortness of breath is called to your attention, it is better to take it seriously than to push it out of your mind. Taking it seriously means seeing a physician. The doctor can then check out whether the shortness of breath is normal or abnormal for you. As with most symptoms, delay in finding out about dyspnea is not wise. If there is something wrong, valuable time may be lost, time during which the chance for effective treatment may pass. If there is *not* something wrong, if you or others around you just have a "low threshold," then finding that out will relieve your mind—and theirs. So, "when in doubt, check it out."

WHAT CAUSES SHORTNESS OF BREATH?

If shortness of breath is a signal of disease, what are the possible problems involved? Well, there are a lot of possibilities—just as there are a lot of causes of pain. For example, anemia (low blood counts) can make people short of breath, and anemia has multiple causes. Being overweight can cause dyspnea, as can certain glandular problems, such as an overactive or underactive thyroid gland. Heart diseases of various types are a frequent cause of shortness of breath—without chest pains or other symptoms that point directly to the heart. But the most common reason for dyspnea, abnormal shortness of breath is lung disease.

All of the causes of shortness of breath can usually be sorted out by having a physician take a careful history, do a complete physical examination, and obtain certain simple laboratory tests: a blood count, a chest x-ray examination, an electrocardiogram, and some simple breathing tests. Sometimes more extensive tests will be needed to find out whether anything is really wrong and, if so, what it is. But the doctor also should take your symptoms seriously, not dismiss them with a statement that you are "getting older" or "slowing down in life." The history and physical examination should be done carefully, and at least the tests mentioned should be performed.

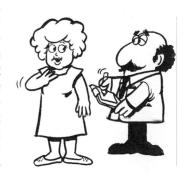

WHAT KINDS OF LUNG DISEASE ARE THERE?

If this sequence has been followed, and if the reason for your shortness of breath turns out to be the most common one—lung disease—you will want to know what kinds of lung diseases there are and what needs to be done to find out what type you have.

There are many diseases that can affect the lungs and lead to shortness of breath. Most of them, particularly the ones with long and complex names, are rare. But despite the many possibilities, lung diseases can be grouped into three main categories: obstructive diseases that make it difficult to expel air from the lungs (reduce air flow and slow down exhalation), restrictive diseases that reduce the volume of the lungs, and diseases that injure and/or block the blood vessels of the lungs.

By far the most common lung diseases are of the obstructive type. That is why the rest of this book is devoted primarily to them. Except for asthma, these diseases—like emphysema and chronic bronchitis—tend to cause shortness of breath, mostly in people beyond age 40. This dyspnea is all too often attributed to "age" or "being out of shape." Therefore, diagnosis is often long delayed because the person does not seek medical attention.

The restrictive diseases cause shortness of breath by either scarring the lungs or filling their air spaces. Usually these diseases are slow and progressive—and so is the shortness of breath they produce. Sometimes the cause of this chronic inflammation and scarring of the lungs is known (e.g., exposure to asbestos, beryllium, or other injurious fumes or particles or an allergic reaction to certain inhaled materials such as cotton dust or pigeon droppings). Such inhalation exposure most often occurs at work, but it may occur at home. Many of the restrictive diseases are of unknown cause. These are grouped under the term *idiopathic*—a terrific medical term that means "of unknown cause." A common form of restrictive lung disease is "idiopathic interstitial pneumonitis." This means the patient has an inflammation of the lung (pneumonitis) that involves the connective tissue of the lung (interstitium) and is of unknown cause. Whether the cause is known or unknown, a diagnosis can be made and a treatment program started. Since scarring may occur, and scars cannot be reversed, an early diagnosis is important—before the scarring and other lung injuries become severe and irreversible.

Diseases of the blood vessels of the lung are less common. They develop because of injury to the small blood vessels in the lung or because blood clots (called emboli) block off the larger pulmonary vessels. Shortness of breath—sometimes developing suddenly, sometimes gradually—is usually the only symptom. Often these diseases go undiagnosed for long periods because patients "adapt" to their breathing limitations and, therefore, feel that nothing is wrong. Again, this is a mistake, because early diagnosis and treatment are vital.

OTHER SIGNS OF LUNG PROBLEMS

Although shortness of breath, at rest or with activity, is the most common signal of lung disease, other problems may come before or after. Among the most frequent are cough, wheezing, chest pains, and coughing up blood.

Cough is, again, something we all experience. It requires your attention if it

- Is persistent. Coughing day after day is not normal.
- Happens without an obvious cause (exposure to fumes; having "the flu").
- Produces yellow or green sputum.

The causes of cough range from sinusitis and chronic bronchitis to more serious things like tumors.

Wheezing—high-pitched whistling sounds coming from your throat or lungs—usually is due to narrowing of your windpipe or bronchial tubes. Lots of people may experience these noises after a virus infection. But if wheezing is persistent, has no obvious cause or is associated with shortness of breath, check it out. The causes range, again, from infections to asthma to tumor.

Having chest pains—of any type—is not normal. However, many kinds of chest pain come from problems that are not serious, such as muscle spasms, heartburn, or minor nerve pinches. But severe chest pains, or ones that persist, mean something—maybe something vital. The causes range widely—from heart attack to virus infections, to blood clots reaching your lungs, to mild rib injuries.

Coughing up blood, clearly, is not normal. If you cough up blood—even "little streaks"—something is wrong. But there are many causes for coughing up blood, ranging from bronchitis and nasal congestion (the most common causes) to malignant tumors. The most common causes are not serious and can be treated easily. But seeing blood in what you cough up means you should act *immediately* to find out *why*.

THE CENTRAL POINTS

This brief summary of the breathing problems and their causes is far from comprehensive. Whole books can be written (and have been!) about any one of them. The central points are these:

- Shortness of breath and other problems may be a signal of disease.
- Determining whether it *is* such a signal ultimately requires evaluation by a doctor.
- Any of the breathing problems listed—if sudden in onset, severe, persistent, and without an obvious cause—should be checked out. Chest pains and coughing up blood need prompt attention.

- A good history, physical examination, and simple laboratory tests can usually tell you and the doctor whether disease is present and, if so, what it is.
- Early diagnosis of all the diseases—including those of the lung—is important because delay in diagnosis means delay in treatment.
- Delay in treatment may lead to irreversible changes in the lungs (and, in some instances, in the heart as well).
- Of the lung diseases that cause shortness of breath, the "obstructive" ones are the most common.

This manual is primarily for persons with obstructive lung diseases, but some parts also apply to people with other kinds of lung diseases. If you have a lung disease other than asthma, chronic bronchitis, or emphysema, your doctor can tell you which parts of the book apply to you and which do not. Don't make a self-diagnosis. Proper understanding of your problem and its treatment begins with establishing a firm diagnosis. That is the doctor's job. Don't try to do it for him or her.

2

The Lungs: How They Are
Put Together and How They Work

To understand your disease, you should know how normal lungs are built and how they work. Then it is easier to recognize what has happened to your lungs, why you get certain symptoms, and what you and your doctor can do to improve these symptoms. Some new vocabulary is involved. If you learn these new words, you will be able to talk with your doctor more easily and not be confused by things he or she says or by articles you may read about lung disease.

HOW THE BODY'S ENGINE RUNS

The human body requires oxygen to burn food as fuel for energy, just as automobile engines need oxygen to burn gasoline or diesel fuel and power plants burn coal, oil, or other fuels. And, just as with other fuels, when the body "burns" oxygen for energy, waste products result; the two major waste products are water and carbon dioxide.

Therefore all of the body's functions depend on delivery of a steady supply of oxygen. Unfortunately, the body cannot store much oxygen. If delivery stops, the body "runs out of gas" within about 5 minutes. So the supply must be continuous, unlike the supply of food or water.

Furthermore, the waste products must be excreted promptly. Getting rid of water presents no problems. If the body retains water, it can still function and, sooner or later, excrete (get rid of) it through the kidneys as urine or through the sweat glands. But if carbon dioxide builds up in the body, it creates acids in the blood. An excess of such acids can impair the function of important organs such as the brain and heart. And a build-up of carbon dioxide can produce such symptoms as headaches, drowsiness, and fatigue.

The lungs are designed to solve the twin problems of continuous oxygen delivery and carbon dioxide removal. They are the only route by which oxygen can be delivered to the body. Acids and carbon dioxide can be excreted by the kidneys, but the lungs get rid of carbon dioxide

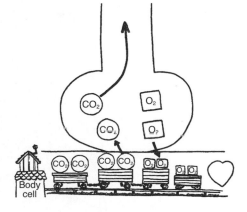

(and prevent acidity) much more quickly and efficiently than do the kidneys.

To carry out these two vital functions, the lungs need to have a practical way to bring fresh air (inspired air) into contact with the blood in a safe manner, so that the blood can pick up oxygen and get rid of excess carbon dioxide. Then the air must be efficiently expelled (expired) into the environment, and the blood pumped to the rest of the body.

HOW THE LUNGS ARE DESIGNED
Step One: Getting Air In and Out

This function is carried out by a system of branching air tubes (bronchial tubes) to bring air in and out of the lungs and a system of blood tubes (pulmonary arteries) to bring blood to the lungs. The system of air tubes is called the *bronchial tree*, an appropriate name because it looks like an upside-down tree. It begins with a single, large tube (like the tree trunk) called the *windpipe* or *trachea*, which you can feel with your fingers in your neck. The trachea extends from the back of the mouth to the inside of the chest (or *thorax*). There, the trachea divides into two major branches (one to the right lung, one to the left lung). Next, each of these main stem bronchi branches many times into smaller and smaller bronchial tubes, just as a tree branches. When the branches become very small (so small that they can be seen only with a microscope), they are given a new name: *bronchioles*. The larger bronchial tubes have cartilage in their walls. Cartilage is a rigid but flexible material—flexible enough to change shape as we breathe but rigid enough to prevent the larger bronchial tubes from collapsing. The smaller bronchial tubes have no cartilage in their walls; they are surrounded by a circle of muscle. If this muscle contracts, the tubes can be narrowed greatly. All bronchial tubes are lined with a delicate layer of cells and lubricating liquid (the *mucous membrane*). Some of the cells in the membrane produce a sticky fluid called *mucus*,

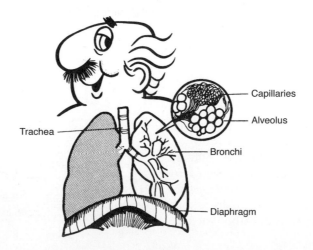

which coats the mucous membrane. Some of the cells also have hairlike structures on them (*cilia*), which beat rhythmically. The mucus lies on top of these cilia—a fact we will talk more about later.

The bronchioles also branch, finally ending in a cluster of little balloon-like structures called the *air sacs* or *alveoli*. There are about 300 million of these alveoli in the lungs. Thus one trachea leads to 300 million alveoli; clearly, that involves a lot of branching! The alveoli have extremely thin walls. They also contain "elastic" tissue in their walls, making them behave much like tiny rubber balloons.

Step Two: Getting Blood In and Out

The system of blood tubes is similar in structure. It begins with one large tube (*main pulmonary artery*) that comes out of the right side of the heart (*right ventricle*). The main artery then splits into a right and a left branch, one supplying each lung. Then each of these branches, like those in the bronchial system, divides many times into smaller and smaller pulmonary arteries. The smallest branches of this system also get a new name: *arterioles*. The arterioles run along the walls of the bronchioles. Finally, the arterioles reach the alveoli; there they divide again into tiny vessels called *capillaries*. The capillaries are in the walls of the alveoli. Therefore, the blood in the capillaries is separated from the air in the alveoli only by the extremely thin, elastic walls of the alveoli. This is why it is normally so easy for oxygen to get into, and carbon dioxide out of, the blood. There are about 1 billion capillaries, more than three for each air sac.

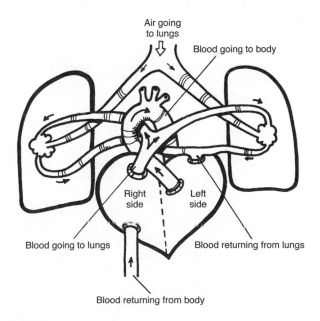

Air going
to lungs

Blood going to body

Right
side

Left
side

Blood going to lungs

Blood returning from lungs

Blood returning from body

Once the blood has passed through the capillaries (and taken up new oxygen and disposed of excess carbon dioxide), it goes to the left side of the heart (*left atrium and ventricle*). The left ventricle now pumps this "fresh" blood to the organs of the body through the arteries. Therefore, the arteries contain blood that has just come from the lungs. If the lungs are working properly, this blood contains a normal amount of oxygen and carbon dioxide; if they are not, the amount of oxygen and carbon dioxide may be abnormal—the oxygen decreased and the carbon dioxide increased. That is why blood is often taken from arteries and analyzed; these *arterial blood gas values* tell your doctor whether your lungs are doing their job.

There is often confusion in people's minds about the "right side" and the "left side" of the heart. Although both sides are in one package (the heart) in your chest, you now know that the right side of the heart pumps blood to the lungs; the left side receives this "fresh" blood and pumps it to the rest of the body. Therefore the right side of the heart can be affected directly by lung diseases. The left side is not. The blood in your arm or leg *veins* is returning to the right heart to be pumped to the lungs. The veins are bluish and do not pulsate. Your arm or leg *arteries* contain blood that has just come from the lungs and is on its way to your organs (brain, kidney, muscles, and so on). The *arteries* usually cannot be seen except as pulsations, but these pulsations are felt easily.

How the "Respiratory Pump" Works

There are a few more things you should know about how the lungs work. For example, what makes air go into (*inspiration*) and out of (*expiration*) the lungs? The elastic lungs are contained within an airtight container, the chest or *thorax*. The chest is sealed at its lower end by the *diaphragm*, a thin muscle that separates the chest from the *abdomen* (stomach cavity). The diaphragm moves up and down like a piston. When it moves down (inspiration), the airtight thorax expands and a slight vacuum (negative pressure) is created. Air from the outside is therefore sucked into the lungs to overcome this vacuum. The elastic alveoli

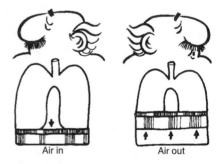

Air in   Air out

are stretched, like expanding balloons. Then the diaphragm relaxes and moves upward. The thorax becomes smaller, as do the elastic alveoli, which—again acting like balloons—expel the air from the lungs. For this system to work, it must be airtight so that a vacuum can be created during breathing. To assure this air tightness, the inner side of the chest wall and the outer side of the lungs are covered with a thin membrane (sheet of cells) called the *pleura*, which is moistened by a tiny amount of fluid so that the lungs slide smoothly as the thorax (chest wall) expands and contracts.

We are usually not aware of these things. Breathing normally goes on without our thinking about it, but, as you know or will learn here, that is not the case if the lungs become abnormal. When the lungs become abnormal, muscles other than the diaphragm may be used to make the thorax larger and smaller. These are the intercostal muscles (between the ribs) and several muscles in the neck called *accessory muscles*. Usually, these muscles have little work to do during breathing, but in lung disease they may have to do a great deal of work in breathing.

What "Controls" Breathing?

There is another thing that most of us do not think about when we breathe. How do we know *how much* to breathe? What controls *how deep* and *how fast* we breathe? Actually, we have a complicated "control" system built into the body that works a lot like a thermostat for regulating a central heating/cooling system. The usual thermostat registers temperature and turns the heater or air conditioner on or off to keep the temperature where you want it. The "breathing thermostat" senses the oxygen and carbon dioxide in the blood. It turns the breathing apparatus on and off (or makes it go faster or slower) to keep oxygen and carbon dioxide in the blood at proper levels. If the oxygen level in the blood falls, or if the carbon dioxide level rises, this "thermostat" makes you breathe harder (more quickly and deeper). That is why, for example, when people go to high altitude, where the amount of oxygen in the air is less, they breathe faster and deeper.

How the Lungs Are Protected

Finally, there are some things you should know about how the lungs protect themselves against impurities and other changes in the air we breathe. As you know, the air around us can be hot or cold or wet or dry and can contain various irritating gases and particles. The lungs are rather delicate and work best when the air in them is *moist*, is at *body temperature* (37°C; 98.6°F), and is free of particles or irritating gases. Nature has designed several "protective" systems so that the lungs receive such air. The first of these systems is the *upper air passages*—the nose, the mouth, and the back of the mouth (*oropharynx*), where air entering the mouth or nose comes together. Above and around the nose and mouth are some "spaces," called *sinuses*, built into the skull. These upper air passages and sinuses have two jobs: to regulate the temperature and the wetness of the air you breathe in and to remove irritating particles and gases from this air. If the system works, air entering your windpipe will be at just the right temperature and wetness and will be free of impurities. Thus the upper air passages can warm or cool inhaled air and can add or remove water from it; furthermore, irritant gases or particles are "trapped" in the mucus that coats these passages and are then removed by cough, sneeze, expectoration, or nose blowing.

If the upper air passages fail or are unable to do these things properly, air enters the lungs in less than optimal condition. The lungs themselves have several protection systems that then swing into action. The mucous membranes of the air tubes also are equipped to warm or cool air and to adjust its wetness. Particles or irritants can be "trapped" in the mucus that coats the bronchial tubes. After they are trapped, they can be coughed out or, more commonly, removed by a "mucus escalator" built into the lungs. There is a real "escalator" in the bronchial tree that consists of the mucous layer, which is propelled from the small tubes to the windpipe by the *cilia* that beat toward the windpipe. This mucus is then either swallowed (without our being aware of it) or coughed out.

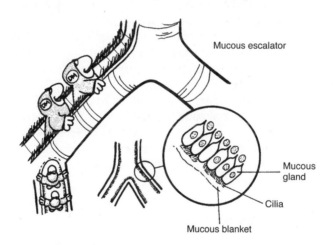

Of course, *cough* is another protection. Cough is produced by irritation of the bronchial tubes. This expels mucus much more rapidly than the "escalator." Cough also may alert us to the fact that we are inhaling irritating things and tell us to move away from them (if possible). Another "protection" is bronchial spasm. With severe irritation, the bronchial muscles contract, even in normal people. This is the body's way of trying to protect us from inhaling irritants (by clamping down the small bronchial tubes). The sensation is an unpleasant one, but it may alert us to an irritant exposure from which we should escape.

Finally, some irritating gases or particles may defy these elaborate protective systems and reach the air sacs. Even then, another defense system exists; this consists of white blood cells of a special kind called *macrophages*. These cells wander through the air sacs searching for debris—viruses, bacteria, particles that were inhaled. They engulf (suck up) such things, carry them off, and digest them. These cells cannot carry away *all* inhaled irritants. Some stay in the lungs and may cause irritation, future scarring, or other problems.

This, then, is the way the normal lungs work and how they are constructed. Knowing about these things should help you to understand how to take care of your lungs and how, when they are injured or abnormal, to help them to work better.

3

COPD: What Does That Mean?

As has already been indicated, there are many lung diseases. The most common type of lung disease is obstructive lung disease. This is often referred to as COPD, which stands for **C**hronic **O**bstructive **P**ulmonary **D**isease. This term refers to a group of diseases that all share one common feature: difficulty in expelling air from the lungs. This is called *expiratory obstruction*.

There are three disease processes that are usually lumped together under the label of COPD: chronic bronchitis, emphysema, and asthma. Although each of these diseases develops in a different way, all cause expiratory obstruction. For patients, distinction among these three disorders is not critical because most persons with COPD have some combination, and many of the symptoms and treatments are the same. (For research purposes, however, distinction among the different kinds of COPD remains important.)

CHRONIC BRONCHITIS

The problem in chronic bronchitis results from chronic inflammation and swelling of the cells lining the inside of the bronchi (air tubes). When inflamed, these cells produce excessive quantities of mucus. The swelling of these cells narrows the air tubes, making breathing more difficult. The excess mucus narrows the tubes further and even blocks some completely. The irritation and excess mucus often cause chronic cough

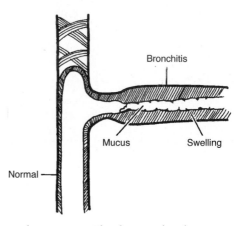

as your body attempts to expectorate the mucus. The lungs also become more easily infected because of these abnormalities. With repeated infections, lung damage may occur. Airways may become permanently dilated (*bronchiectasis*). Alveoli may become scarred (*fibrosis*). The narrowing of the bronchial tubes makes it more difficult for air to move in and out of them. If some tubes become blocked with mucus, the air sacs they supply cannot receive oxygen or get rid of carbon dioxide; they may, at least temporarily, collapse.

EMPHYSEMA

Emphysema is a disease in which the walls of the alveoli (air sacs) fracture (break). As these walls rupture, one larger air sac replaces two, four, or many more small ones. The result is that the number of air sacs (alveoli) is reduced and many of those that remain are enlarged. One large sac is less elastic than the many tiny sacs were. Thus the patient with emphysema has lungs of *reduced elasticity*. To visualize the problems this causes, think of how a balloon works. You must blow air in (work) to fill it. But when you stop blowing, the balloon recoils (deflates) without your doing anything. The balloon's own elasticity causes it to expel the air. This is how normal lungs work. You must work to inflate your lungs with air (inspire). But when you relax, the lungs recoil (deflate) without effort on your part. Normal expiration (blowing air out of the lungs) is, therefore, a passive event. It just happens.

In a person with emphysema the lungs and alveoli behave more like a paper bag. When you blow air into a paper bag, then stop blowing, what happens? Nothing. The bag stays full of air because it is nonelastic; it does not recoil. To empty the air from a paper bag, you must squeeze it out—and you must expend effort to push the air out. People with emphysema must do the same thing: expend energy during expiration to squeeze air out of the lungs.

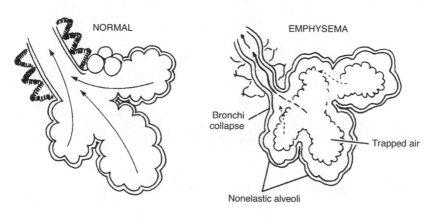

Furthermore, this loss of lung elasticity affects the smaller bronchial tubes. To push air out of these less elastic lungs, a higher pressure must be developed inside the chest. This higher pressure tends to collapse the smaller bronchial tubes, making it even harder to empty air from the alveoli. Worse expiratory obstruction results as the "neck of the balloon" (the bronchial tube) becomes narrowed. This tendency of the bronchial tubes to collapse also occurs with cough and makes it more difficult for the patient to cough up mucus. This collection of mucus, in turn, makes the lungs more susceptible to infection.

ASTHMA

The problem in asthma is that some irritant makes the muscles of the bronchial tubes go into spasm. This spasm narrows the bronchial tubes. Often this same irritant inflames the lining cells of the bronchial tubes, causing them to swell and increase their production of mucus (secretions). These changes further narrow and clog up the bronchial tubes. When these things happen, the patient notices shortness of breath and sometimes cough and wheezing (a whistling sound in the chest).

There are several irritants that produce asthma. One is an *allergen*; that is, some material to which the patient is allergic. An allergy can show up as a skin rash, as an upset stomach, or as bronchial spasm (asthma). Infection is another source of irritation (inflammation), as are cold air, smog, and cigarette smoke.

Many persons with asthma have bronchial muscle that is more irritable than normal. Therefore, small amounts of inhaled irritants can cause bronchial spasm in them, but not in other people. This "hyperirritability" of the bronchial tubes may run in families (that is, it may be inherited).

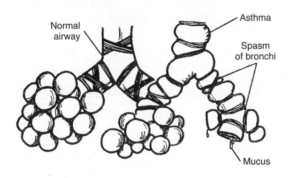

COPD: HOW DO YOU GET IT?

The causes of chronic obstructive lung disease have not been definitely determined. It is likely that the causes of emphysema, chronic bronchitis, and asthma are quite different. However, some features are common to each. For example, heredity seems to play a role in the tendency to develop each disorder.

Air pollution, occupational exposure to dust and fumes, and lung infections make all forms of COPD worse. Allergy plays a role in some people with asthma but not in emphysema or bronchitis. Most of these things cannot be controlled by the affected person. But one factor is under the individual's control: *cigarette smoking*. Emphysema and chronic bronchitis rarely develop in nonsmokers; asthma is worsened by cigarette smoking.

COPD: WHAT ARE THE SYMPTOMS?

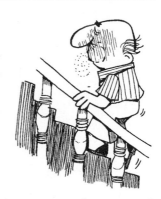

Usually the first thing a person with emphysema notices is difficult breathing—shortness of breath—on exertion (as when climbing stairs or walking quickly). As noted in Chapter 1, this symptom is often disregarded, and the person thinks it just means he or she is "out of shape" or "getting older." The first symptoms of chronic bronchitis are cough and mucus production. These symptoms are like a "chest cold" that hangs on week after week. Later, shortness of breath on exertion develops. The cough, mucus (sputum) production, and shortness of breath all may become suddenly worse if the patient has the "flu" or some other type of lung infection.

Asthma usually starts with rather sudden attacks of cough, shortness of breath, and wheezing. These attacks may come and go at first. Many persons with asthma have normal or near-normal lung function in between episodes. Later on, in some persons, cough, mild wheezing, and shortness of breath may be present all the time (i.e., become "chronic"). The attacks may come on more frequently at certain times of the year (particularly spring or fall), after exposure to known allergens or irritants, only during exercise, or with the onset of a "cold." However, wheezing attacks also may appear without an obvious cause.

COPD: HOW DO YOU KNOW YOU HAVE IT?

The diagnosis of COPD involves many factors. The first step is for you to consult your doctor if you have any of the symptoms of COPD. The most common symptom is shortness of breath, particularly on exertion (walking up steps, carrying packages, hurrying during level walking). Affected persons often first notice that they "can't keep up with" their spouses or friends. A chronic cough and wheezing may be other symptoms. However, problems *other than* COPD can cause similar symptoms. Trouble breathing, like pain in the chest, can mean many different things.

Your doctor will perform a physical examination and other tests as needed. The physical examination will include examining your chest and listening to your breath sounds with a stethoscope. People with emphysema have excess air in the lungs, making their lungs and chest larger than normal and causing breath sounds to be more "quiet" and "distant." An x-ray picture of the chest can be taken to help this evaluation, but it cannot be used alone to diagnose COPD or other causes of lung symptoms.

Pulmonary (lung) function tests are useful for determining whether you have COPD or some other problem. These involve breathing into one or

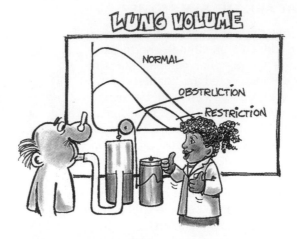

more machines that measure how well your lungs are working. The simplest test, called spirometry, can be performed in a doctor's office or laboratory and measures the flow of air into and out of the lungs. Your test results are compared with "normal" standards based on your age, height, gender, race, and weight. Other, more complex pulmonary function tests are performed in a laboratory. These may be used to measure the volume of air in the lungs or the efficiency of the lungs in exchanging gas (i.e., oxygen and carbon dioxide) with the air. They can help your doctor confirm your diagnosis and more accurately estimate the severity of your disease. The information can also be used to help determine eligibility for disability or a handicap parking permit.

Another useful test involves obtaining a small blood sample from an artery (arterial blood gas) at rest and/or during exercise to determine how well the lungs are delivering oxygen to the blood and removing carbon dioxide from it. Oximetry is another test commonly used to determine the oxygen saturation level in the blood. This test uses a small probe that shines light through the skin (e.g., through a finger or ear). Although easier and not as invasive as an arterial blood gas measurement, it is less accurate and does not provide information about the carbon dioxide level. These tests are very important for determining your need for treatment with oxygen to restore a low blood oxygen level to a more normal range. For patients with lung disease, supplemental oxygen is just like any other drug. Its proper use requires careful assessment of whether you need it (not everyone with lung disease does) and how much you need.

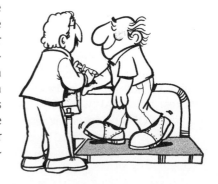

The body's need for oxygen is greater with exercise than at rest. An exercise test, which may involve walking on a treadmill or cycling on a stationary bicycle, allows your physician to assess your capacity for physical activity and your body's response to exercise, including any changes in oxygen or carbon dioxide levels in the blood.

Using this evaluation as a basis, your doctor can determine whether you have COPD or another condition that causes shortness of breath and then develop a proper treatment plan designed for you. No matter which kind of lung disease you have, the physical examination, chest x-ray, pulmonary function tests, and blood gas measurements provide valuable information.

COPD: WHAT CAN BE DONE ABOUT IT?

The most important factor in your treatment will be the relationship you have with your doctor. You must be willing to be frank and honest, and your doctor must be the same with you. Some parts of your treatment, such as prescribing drugs, treatment, tests, and diets, will be the doctor's responsibility. A big responsibility is yours. You must take the medicines as ordered, do your treatments at home, practice proper breathing, eat correctly, and, most important of all, quit smoking if you haven't already. The treatment of COPD is a cooperative venture.

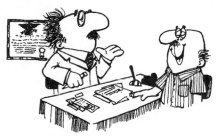

Each person's disease is different. Only your doctor knows which treatments and therapies are right for you. But only you know how you feel and how you respond to various treatments. Work with your doctor; ask questions. The more you know about your disease, the better off you are. The more your doctor knows about you, the better the treatment program that can be planned for you.

The treatment of COPD may include some or all of the following:

- Medications
- Good hydration (fluid intake)
- Proper breathing techniques
- Adequate diet
- Use of respiratory therapy
- Maintenance of muscle tone
- Graded physical activity
- Prevention and treatment of infections
- Use of supplemental oxygen in some cases
- Weight control
- Avoidance of allergens and/or irritants
- Bronchial drainage to remove excess mucus

The precise nature of your condition will determine the type of treatment prescribed. Sometimes very limited medication is all that is needed. Sometimes rather extensive treatment is required. The aims of treatment are to reverse the reversible, to preserve the function you have, to prevent complications, and to teach you how to use the function that you have more efficiently. These aims can be achieved whether your problem is mild or severe.

COPD: WHAT IS YOUR RESPONSIBILITY?

Now that you have an understanding of what COPD means and the goals of treatment, it's time to add the most important ingredient—*you*. With enthusiasm, perseverance, and knowledge, you can play a big role in controlling your disease and alleviating some of your symptoms. The remainder of this manual is devoted to all aspects of treatment. After your doctor has outlined the various therapies he or she wants you to use, consult your manual for guidance and review.

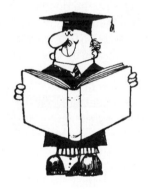

4

Understanding Your Medications

Many people with lung disease take medications to improve their breathing and feel better. It is important to ask why the medication is prescribed, exactly how to take it, and what positive or negative reactions may occur. People are often afraid to take certain medications—and thus secretly don't take them. That is not in their best interest. Friends, relatives, and people without medical training dispense a lot of wrong information. Discuss each medicine with your doctor or pharmacist, both of whom can give you good information about all medications. Bring an updated list of all your medications to each doctor's appointment.

To treat the various types of lung diseases, different medications are used. Each medicine does a specific job to help the lungs function more effectively. Your doctor will determine which medications you need on the basis of your history, the physical examination, the results of breathing tests, and other laboratory studies.

All medicines are chemicals. They may come from plant sources or from animals. Synthesized drugs are entirely human made. Medicines have their beneficial effects, but they may cause side effects. A medicine taken by mouth must enter the stomach and then the blood in order to reach the lungs. Not only can medicines upset the stomach, but also they pass through many other organs while on their way to the lungs and may exert these other effects, called side effects. Most of the time these effects are well tolerated and may disappear with time. You should be familiar with what your medicine is supposed to do and also with its side effects.

Another important fact to remember is that each medicine has two names: a generic (chemical) name and a brand (company) name. The generic name is always the same for each drug, no matter which company manufactures it. The brand name for a drug is the property of the company that markets that drug. In some states it is possible for your pharmacist to substitute a less expensive generic brand drug for the more expensive branded product. Sometimes this practice may cause you some confusion, and you may think you have received the wrong prescription. If you have any questions because the pills look different to you, consult with your pharmacist. Besides providing you with medicines, many pharmacies provide other helpful services. For example, many pharmacists maintain a complete record of all prescriptions you have received from any physician, dentist, or other doctor. This "patient profile" can then be reviewed periodically by the pharmacist for drug interactions, a situation that occurs when two or more drugs taken at the same time work against each other. Ask your pharmacist or physician to explain this in more detail.

For each category of medication that follows, list (with the help of your physician, pharmacist, or nurse) the names of the medications you take, along with the dose's desired effect and potential side effects, and the time schedule for each drug.

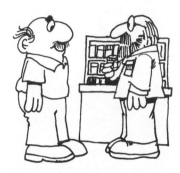

BRONCHODILATORS (Open Up Your Airways)

Bronchodilators relax the muscles of the breathing tubes, making them wider and allowing air to get in and out more easily. Bronchodilators can be taken as pills, liquids, or aerosol sprays (see Chapter 5). The most common of these drugs are adrenergic (adrenaline-like) drugs, anticholinergic (atropine-like) drugs, and theophylline (a xanthine). There are many different preparations of these types of drugs, and new ones appear regularly. Newer medications tend to be safer, easier to use, and more selective in their effects. As with all medicines, there may be side effects. Xanthine drugs may cause an upset stomach and heartburn. Adrenergic drugs, depending on the form taken (pill or spray) and on how much you use, can increase your heart rate, make you feel jittery or nervous, or cause muscle tremors. Delivering adrenergic and anticholinergic drugs in metered dose inhalers results in the best desired effects on the smooth muscle with the least side effects.

STEROIDS (Anti-inflammatory)

Steroid drugs are all "relatives" of the hormone *cortisol*, which the body produces normally. These corticosteroids help to dilate the bronchial tubes, decrease the swelling of bronchial tube lining, and decrease lung inflammation. Steroids also have many potential side effects. They may make you feel very energetic and give you a (false) sense of well-being. Other common side effects include weight gain, redistribution of fat, easy bruising, stomach irritation, diabetes, and cataracts in the eyes. The side effects depend on the dose of the drug taken, how you take it (pill or spray), and the length of time you take it. You must never discontinue oral steroids yourself or alter the dose without your physician's advice. Abrupt withdrawal of steroids can be life threatening because your body has temporarily lost its ability to make natural steroids. People often hear stories about the side effects of steroids—stories that worry them. Remember that the side effects relate to the amount and the time schedule of any drug you take. Steroids are no different. And, like any drug, your doctor prescribes them only when you need them and in the amounts you require. For many years, steroids were available only by pill or injection. Now certain special steroids can be inhaled as an aerosol, directly into the lungs. Inhaled steroids are absorbed very slowly and poorly into the blood. Therefore they have beneficial effects on the lungs while causing fewer side effects. For people who need only small doses of steroids, these inhalations may replace oral steroids. Steroids taken by oral inhalation can cause oral thrush. Rinsing your mouth after each use may help prevent this. However, all steroids must be taken on a regular schedule because they do not give immediate effects; so they are not to be used as you "need" them, but regularly, to *prevent* symptoms. Remember, these are potent medicines and must be taken only as directed by your physician.

CROMOLYN SODIUM

Cromolyn sodium is a medication used mainly by patients who have asthma. It is taken by inhalation and works only to *prevent* symptoms and bronchospasm. To do this, it must be taken regularly. It should never be used during an asthmatic attack, because it can actually make an attack worse. Another drug in this category is Nedocromil, which also inhibits activation of inflammatory cells.

DIGITALIS

Digitalis is the generic, overall name for heart pills that strengthen the heart muscle. These drugs make the heart beat more slowly and with more force. Most patients with lung disease do not have heart problems that require digitalis, but some do. Digitalis drugs must be used carefully. The dose should never be changed without your doctor's order.

EXPECTORANTS

The purpose of expectorants is to liquefy secretions and make them easier to cough up. Generally, only patients with very heavy bronchial secretions use them. Their value is debated, with no conclusive medical opinion as to whether or not they work. The most widely used expectorants are potassium iodide (SSKI) and glycerol guaiacolate (GG). Potassium iodide can cause a rash and swelling of the salivary glands because of allergies to iodide. Newer types of expectorants have been developed and are being evaluated. Drinking adequate water and staying well hydrated is the most effective way to keep secretions liquid.

ANTIBIOTICS

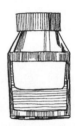

Antibiotic medications are used to help fight bacterial infections. There are many different types that are used against different bacteria. Some are given as pills or capsules, others by injection. Penicillin, sulfa drugs, tetracycline, and erythromycin are generic names of some of the drugs in this category that are commonly used for patients with lung diseases. You should take these drugs in the exact dose and at the time specified by your doctor, who will tell you what side effects may occur. For example, an upset stomach or bowel problems are common side effects with certain antibiotics. It is important to know when and how antibiotics should be taken. Some antibiotics should be taken between meals because food may interfere with drug absorption, whereas others should be taken with meals to prevent stomach upset. You must always finish the course of antibiotic therapy that your physician prescribes, even when you feel better after only a few doses. When you get your prescription filled, remind your doctor or pharmacist of any allergies you may have to antibiotics.

DIURETICS

Diuretics (water pills) help rid your body of excess fluid. This fluid retention, called *edema*, usually shows up as swollen ankles and legs. There are many reasons that edema may develop in patients with lung disease. Your doctor will provide you with guidelines on the use of the drugs that treat edema. Overuse of diuretics can make you weak and should be avoided (see Potassium Supplements).

POTASSIUM SUPPLEMENTS

When diuretics are taken regularly, they cause loss of not only fluid but also potassium. This may result in weakness and leg cramps. Potassium supplements are given to counteract these effects. Eating high-potassium foods is sometimes sufficient to replenish lost potassium (see Chapter 11).

MOOD ELEVATORS

Mood elevating drugs are designed to help you feel less depressed. People with chronic health problems often have periods of feeling "blue." If this feeling persists, you should consult your doctor or a psychiatrist for help in dealing with this problem.

TRANQUILIZERS AND SEDATIVES

Tranquilizers and sedatives are designed to calm or relax you and to help you sleep. These drugs can dangerously depress your breathing if taken in excess. Never increase the dose without consulting your doctor. Some symptoms (such as insomnia or irritability) may mean that your lungs are not working properly and that sedatives and tranquilizers should be decreased, not increased. Your physician knows when and how to adjust the dose of these drugs.

FLU AND PNEUMONIA VACCINES

Vaccines help you to fight off serious viral (flu) infections and certain bacterial (pneumococcal) infections. A new flu vaccine is prepared each year and is usually available in the fall before the start of the flu season. The pneumococcal vaccine needs to be given only once every 5 to 10 years.

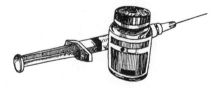

OXYGEN

Sometimes patients with lung disease cannot transfer enough oxygen from the alveoli to the blood; therefore the amount of oxygen in the blood falls below normal levels. A low blood oxygen level impairs the body's engine (see Chapter 2). Whatever the reason for the oxygen lack, the treatment is the same: take a drug that overcomes the deficiency. In the case of oxygen deficit, that "drug" is oxygen.

Like all drugs, oxygen is prescribed by your doctor. Your doctor orders the drugs you take for your respiratory problem in a specific amount, at specific times, by a specific route. For example, aminophylline (drug), 250 mg (dose), four times a day (times), by mouth (route). Likewise, your doctor prescribes oxygen in the same manner: oxygen (drug), 2 liters/minute (dose), during exercise (time), by nasal cannula (route). Your doctor determines the appropriate dose based on blood oxygen level measurements taken at rest and while exercising. As with other drugs, you must not increase or decrease your oxygen flow without the doctor's advice. Turning the liter flow above the prescribed dose may cause serious complications.

Remember that millions of dollars each year are spent on medicines. You can help make the most of your medicine dollars by taking your medications as prescribed and by communicating problems with your doctor.

5

Respiratory Therapy: What Oxygen and Aerosols Can Do for You

Getting air into and out of the lungs is what breathing is all about. Getting oxygen from the air to the cells in the body to burn fuel and create energy is how living things survive. Most people take breathing and oxygen for granted, until something prevents them from breathing easily or from having enough oxygen to fuel their body's needs.

Many people with chronic lung diseases can benefit from the use of various respiratory therapy techniques. Aerosol medications used in metered dose inhalers or in breathing machines can help make difficult breathing easier. Techniques of bronchial hygiene can be used to aid in removing excess mucus from the lungs. In persons with low blood oxygen levels, supplemental oxygen can be used to restore oxygen levels to a safer and more normal range. During an emergency room visit or a stay in the hospital, most people with chronic lung disease will be treated with some type of respiratory therapy or equipment. These topics are typically covered in some detail during a pulmonary rehabilitation program.

Respiratory therapy equipment comes in various sizes, complexities, and costs. The indications and prescription for treatments and/or equipment should be determined by your physician. A respiratory therapist, nurse, or home medical equipment supply company can help you to select the right device and to better understand the proper use and care of your equipment.

Individual needs vary greatly; there is no single treatment plan or piece of equipment that is right for everyone with chronic lung disease. The device that gave you so much relief in the hospital or in the doctor's office may present some problems for you at home and may not be the best choice there. You can also learn and practice respiratory care techniques that help your breathing more than a machine can. There is no substitute for being informed about your disease.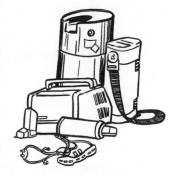

If you do need equipment at home, the simplest device that will do the job is the best choice. **Remember: The more complex the equipment, the bigger your commitment is for its use, care, and maintenance.** To achieve maximal benefits, you should clearly understand the purpose, correct usage, and maintenance of the equipment prescribed for you.

Also, remember that cost is not always a good measure of the value of a device. Inexpensive devices are often as effective as costly ones. Fancy dials and gadgets are no indication that you are getting "the best." Your doctor, respiratory therapist, or nurse should be familiar with these devices and will indicate whether you need them and which best suits your condition.

The devices most frequently used for home care can be conveniently grouped into two categories: oxygen therapy and aerosol therapy. This chapter describes the equipment associated with the delivery of oxygen as "oxygen therapy equipment" and the devices that produce visible mist for inhalation as "aerosol therapy equipment." You may need a combination of these treatments.

OXYGEN THERAPY

What is oxygen? It is an atmospheric element essential for life, a gas, and a drug. Every cell in the body needs energy to function. Cells get their energy from a combination (metabolism) of the food we eat plus oxygen. This energy enables us to carry out all bodily functions, such as using our muscles to breathe and to perform work.

The air that we breathe contains approximately 21% oxygen. It is inhaled and travels through air passages to alveoli (air sacs) in the lungs, where the oxygen is mixed with the blood in small blood vessels called capillaries. The oxygen attaches to the hemoglobin in the red blood cells in the blood; the heart then pumps the oxygen-rich blood to parts of the body. Carbon dioxide is a gas that is produced as a waste product by the cells in the act of creating energy, during metabolism. It is circulated in the blood, back to the lungs, and eliminated from our bodies as we exhale. This process by which the body takes in oxygen and eliminates carbon dioxide is called *gas exchange*. If gas exchange does not occur normally, the level of oxygen and carbon dioxide in your blood can become unbalanced. Lung function, heart function, and blood and hemoglobin levels all have an impact on gas exchange. There are many reasons that some people with chronic lung disease have low oxygen levels while others do not. For example, airway diseases such as asthma and bronchitis can limit airflow into and out of the lungs. Emphysema causes loss of elasticity in the lung and damages or destroys alveoli. In these diseases, air may not flow well to all areas, or it may become trapped and "stale." When this happens, the lungs may not be able to completely replenish the oxygen or remove the excess carbon dioxide from the blood in the capillaries. Then the blood that is pumped to the rest of the body will be low in oxygen and/or high in carbon dioxide. Some people with low blood oxygen levels may show signs of blue nail beds, ears, nose, or lips. Often, however, there are no visible signs, which is why an assessment by your physician is so important.

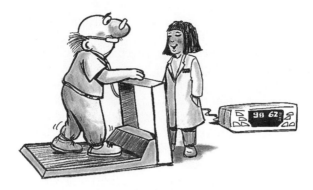

Blood oxygen levels are assessed by two methods: *oximetry* and *arterial blood gases* (ABGs). Oximetry involves the use of a device with a light and a sensor that can be placed over the finger or the ear lobe to measure oxygen saturation indirectly. This is done by analyzing the transmission of light through the capillary bed under the skin. This method is helpful for monitoring trends in blood oxygen levels without obtaining a blood sample. Oximetry can be used in doctors' offices, clinics, the gym, and your home. The other method of assessing blood oxygen level is measurement of arterial blood gases, which involves drawing blood directly from an artery, often in the wrist area. Specially maintained equipment and trained technicians are needed to obtain and process the blood sample. This method tends to be more accurate and provides additional important information, such as the carbon dioxide level in the blood. However, it is more difficult, less convenient, and more expensive than oximetry.

Oxygen therapy may be prescribed when one of these tests shows a low blood oxygen level and demonstrates the medical need for treatment with supplemental oxygen. Oxygen therapy is **NOT** prescribed just to treat shortness of breath or fatigue. There are many reasons that patients with chronic lung disease can become short of breath without having low oxygen levels. No recommended standard exists for how often an arterial blood gas or oximetry test should be performed. This is at the discretion of your physician. However, many health insurers require an annual test to continue coverage for oxygen prescriptions.

What if your body is not getting enough oxygen? It is known that blood vessels often constrict (narrow) when oxygen levels are low. The right side of the heart must work harder to pump blood through these narrowed blood vessels. The result can be an increased strain on the right side of the heart. This strain can be reduced by increasing the available oxygen in the blood and using supplemental oxygen as prescribed. Medical studies have shown that people with low blood oxygen levels live longer and better lives if they use oxygen than if they do not.

If your blood oxygen level is low, your physician will prescribe supplemental oxygen for you. Used in treatment, oxygen is considered a drug. As with any other drug, it is essential to have a prescription for oxygen. The prescription should tell you when to use oxygen and how much to use. Many people with chronic lung disease may have prescriptions that direct them to use one amount of oxygen at rest and during sleep and a higher amount with physical activity. Others use oxygen only with activity or sleep or when going to a higher altitude. It is important to keep in mind that being out of breath does not necessarily mean that you have a low blood oxygen level. The only way to be certain is to be assessed by medical professionals with an arterial blood gas or oximetry test, preferably both at rest and with exertion.

Oxygen makes up 21% of the air around us. Oxygen for medical treatment can be extracted from the air by very special industrial processes that yield 100% oxygen that has been purified and dehumidified. Once extracted, oxygen can be packaged commercially and made available for home delivery as a compressed gas or by freezing it into a liquid. In addition, there are devices for the home that run on electricity and can concentrate oxygen in the air.

A wide variety of oxygen systems are available for home use. Both stationary and portable respiratory equipment can be rented or purchased. The choice of oxygen sources for the home is broader than ever before and continues to improve. Your respiratory therapist, nurse, or home equipment vendor can assist you in finding the correct pieces of equipment to fit your lifestyle and needs.

OXYGEN EQUIPMENT

Sources of Oxygen

Oxygen is produced by a process of distilling out water vapor and impurities from atmospheric air. The air is separated into the various gases; pure oxygen is then packaged into either compressed gas tanks/cylinders or chilled into a liquid form and stored in a thermos-like reservoir. A third way that oxygen can be supplied for home use is by an oxygen concentrator.

COMPRESSED GAS: TANKS AND CYLINDERS

The most common and oldest method for storing oxygen is by compression of the gas into an aluminum or steel cylinder at approximately 2300 to 2500 pounds above atmospheric pressure. Tanks come in many sizes. Large stationary ones are often placed in the home, sometimes as backup for another type of system; smaller tanks may be used for physical activities in and around the home, exercise, or travel outside the home. The weight of a portable system is an important factor in determining its portability. For safety reasons, full, high-pressure cylinders must be secured upright in a stand or cart that is supplied with the oxygen.

LIQUID OXYGEN

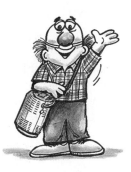

Liquid oxygen is widely used for people who lead active lifestyles. Oxygen is changed from a gas into a liquid form by freezing it to 300 degrees below zero and storing it in a thermos-like reservoir. The advantages of liquid oxygen are that it takes up less space than the gas form, so that more oxygen can be stored in a smaller space. You can then fill a portable reservoir when you are ready to leave home. However, it cannot be stored for long periods of time because it "evaporates" as it is warmed and becomes a gas again. When the gas pressure rises inside the liquid oxygen system, gas is released (vented) to the outside. Liquid oxygen is extremely cold and can spill like any other liquid; therefore, caution in handling is required.

OXYGEN CONCENTRATOR

Thanks to space program technology, electrical devices that extract and concentrate oxygen from room air are also available. An oxygen concentrator is an electrical unit about the size of a nightstand or an end table. The concentrator "makes its own oxygen" from room air by filtering, collecting, and concentrating the oxygen molecules, which are then delivered at your prescribed liter flow. Advantages of this method of oxygen therapy are that it does not require refilling or replacing of tanks, it is not a dry gas, it can be easier to manage, and it may be less expensive over the long run. However, there are also disadvantages. Oxygen concentrators are not very portable, which means that if you are using oxygen 24 hours a day, a portable system such as a small oxygen tank will be needed for use outside your home. With the newest technology, oxygen concentrators can now fill a small portable compressed gas oxygen cylinder in the home. Use of an oxygen concentrator may also increase your electric bill (although most gas and electric companies offer reduced rates for life-supporting equipment, provided you register with them); it also may be noisy and give off heat. Back-up cylinders are required in the event of a power failure. If you use a high flow rate, this method may not be adequate because the actual percentage of oxygen inspired may drop as the flow rate increases. It is also very important to have your equipment company verify correct flow and oxygen content during regular periodic maintenance checks. Otherwise, the device may continue to run with air flowing but with lower oxygen levels than you need.

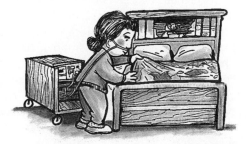

Safety

Oxygen is a relatively safe gas, but it must be handled with caution. Oxygen itself does not burn, but it aids in igniting and speeds burning of combustible/burnable materials. For example, any spark or open flame expands considerably around oxygen, like a "flash-fire." Also, oxygen in tanks is under high pressure; therefore, if the tank is damaged or the top is knocked loose, the tank can "take off" like a rocket or a ruptured balloon. Liquid oxygen is very cold; touching the "frost" that may escape can cause a "frostbite burn."

Storage

- The room in which oxygen is stored should be dry, cool, and well ventilated.
- Keep at least 10 feet between the oxygen source and any possible source of electrical sparks, open flame, or other heat source. Do not permit grease, oil, any other petroleum product, or potentially combustible substances to come into contact or be stored with oxygen equipment. Never smoke or permit anyone to smoke near an oxygen source. Be certain that the oxygen tank is fastened securely. This will prevent it from being knocked over and damaged.
- Avoid inhaling the irritating debris that may accumulate at the bottom of cylinders by changing cylinders when the pressure regulator gauge reads 500 psi (pounds per square inch).

Oxygen Delivery Devices

NASAL CANNULA

The most commonly used appliance for the delivery of low concentrations of oxygen is a nasal cannula. The cannula is a hollow, light plastic tube connected to your oxygen delivery device. It has two small "prong" extensions; one prong enters each nostril. The cannula is kept in place by looping the attached tubing over the ears.

TRANSTRACHEAL CATHETER

Transtracheal oxygen is a relatively new method of delivering oxygen in a more efficient manner. A very thin, unobtrusive catheter is placed directly into the windpipe (trachea) through a small incision in the neck. This is usually done as a minor outpatient surgical procedure. Since oxygen is delivered directly into the trachea, rather than through the nose, the flow rate of oxygen needed can frequently be reduced. This allows 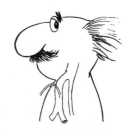 the oxygen source to last longer, a distinct advantage for portable systems. In addition, better oxygenation can be achieved for persons who require high flow rates (4 liters per minute or more). Other possible advantages include more continuous therapy (the catheter stays in place at all times), more comfort and convenience, better cosmetic appearance, and fewer problems related to having the nasal cannula on the face. However, use of the transtracheal catheter also requires regular, fastidious care and cleaning and more problem solving by the patient and caregivers. Appropriate training must be provided.

OXYGEN CONSERVING DEVICES

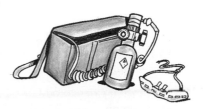

In addition to transtracheal oxygen therapy, other devices have been developed to reduce the oxygen flow requirement and extend the period of time a particular gas source will last. "Reservoir" cannulas provide for storage of oxygen during exhalation in reservoirs located either near the nasal prongs or in a pendant located around the neck. Other devices, called "demand" flow devices, can either be attached to the oxygen source or built into the system. Demand devices turn the flow of oxygen *on* with inspiration (when you "demand" it) and *off* with exhalation, so that oxygen is "conserved" rather than wasted by flowing continuously. Monitoring blood oxygen saturation at rest and during exertion will help determine which piece of equipment is right for you.

ADDITIONAL EQUIPMENT FOR OXYGEN THERAPY

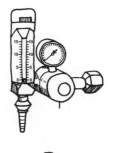

A *regulator* and a *flowmeter* are devices attached to a compressed gas cylinder. The regulator reduces the high pressure of the oxygen as it leaves the cylinder. A dial on the regulator tells you how much compressed gas under pressure is in the cylinder; a full tank of oxygen usually is at about 2200 pounds per square inch (psi) of pressure. As you use the oxygen, the pressure reading will decrease. The regulator and flowmeter are built into a liquid oxygen reservoir. A built-in "fish" scale or contents dial is used to indicate the fullness of a liquid oxygen system. The flowmeter is a measuring device and indicator. It is used to adjust the amount of oxygen that is delivered to you, in liters per minute, as prescribed by your physician. A flowmeter is paired with a regulator if you are using a compressed gas tank or is attached to your liquid oxygen reservoir or oxygen concentrator. It is not safe to use oxygen without flow control.

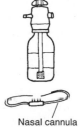

Nasal cannula

A humidifier is a container filled with water and attached to an oxygen flowmeter or other airflow device. The purpose of the humidifier is to add water vapor to the dry oxygen gas.

Myths and Truths About Oxygen

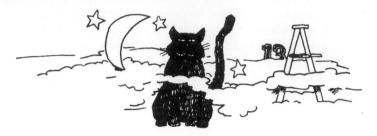

MYTH: Oxygen is flammable.

TRUTH: Oxygen itself DOES NOT BURN. It supports combustion and causes things that do burn to burn faster and hotter.

MYTH: Oxygen can explode.

TRUTH: Oxygen alone IS NOT EXPLOSIVE. Compressed gas cylinders are under a great deal of pressure. If the tank is overfilled, damaged, or ruptured, the gas pressure can cause the cylinder to "pop" or "explode" like a balloon. Oxygen combined with other chemical or gaseous substances can become explosive.

MYTH: Oxygen is addicting. Once you start it, you will have to use it forever.

TRUTH: Oxygen is not addicting. Supplemental oxygen is needed only when your own lungs cannot supply enough. If you no longer need it, you can stop using it.

MYTH: If a little oxygen is good, a lot of oxygen is better.

TRUTH: Oxygen is a drug. Use it only as instructed. As with any other drug, too much can be harmful.

MYTH: Shortness of breath means lack of oxygen. If you become short of breath, you should take oxygen.

TRUTH: Shortness of breath is not always associated with a lack of oxygen. There are many other causes for shortness of breath. Working hard to breathe, as can occur in many chronic lung diseases, can make you short of breath, even if there is plenty of oxygen in your blood. Only by testing the level of oxygen in your blood can your doctor tell if you need supplemental oxygen.

MYTH: People who need to use oxygen must be confined to their homes and can't do anything.

TRUTH: People who use oxygen can lead a normal life. Several types of portable oxygen systems are available. With good planning, you can be active and mobile.

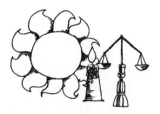

Think Ahead:
Things to Consider Before You Select a Home Oxygen System

1. Ask your doctor, respiratory therapist, or nurse to recommend a practical system for your needs and lifestyle.

2. Ask your doctor, therapist, or nurse to refer you to a reputable medical equipment supplier.

3. Compare portable systems for cost, weight, size, duration of oxygen supply, and refilling capabilities.

4. Evaluate and try several systems to find the product that fits your lifestyle and abilities.

5. Ask a family member or friend to assist you in making the equipment selection and in learning about its use and safety.

6. Be sure that the system you select can meet your body's need for oxygen with exertion as well as at rest.

7. If an oxygen concentrator is recommended, compare size, noise levels, and monthly electricity cost. Ask about newer concentrators that can be used to fill portable cylinders. If you use a concentrator, be sure to register with your gas and electric company for reduced utility rates, if available.

8. Find out whether the system you select is approved by your medical insurance carrier and whether you will be reimbursed for all or part of the cost. The medical equipment company can often assist you.

9. Obtain written instructions from your physician or equipment supplier for the correct use of your oxygen system. Make sure you understand these instructions and are able to easily use the system provided.

10. Learn how to determine the number of hours of oxygen each source will provide. Plan ahead. Arrange deliveries on a regular schedule so you won't run out at night or during a weekend. Keep enough on hand for regular use and have a "back-up" system available for use when there are delivery problems or power outages or in the event of a natural disaster.

AEROSOL THERAPY

Aerosol therapy involves use of respiratory therapy equipment that produces an aerosol or "mist." Inhaling medications in an aerosol is a relatively fast and reliable method of relieving, controlling, or preventing symptoms. Chest infections, congestion with thick secretions, and wheezing may be improved with the inhalation of appropriate medications.

The following information and instructions about the proper use, care, and cleansing of inhaled aerosol medications and their delivery devices can assist you in maintaining relaxed, clear, and open airways in the face of breathing difficulties and infections.

Inhaled aerosol therapy consists of inhaling atomized particles of medications (and possibly a delivery solution) suspended in air directly into the lungs. There are several advantages to delivering medications by inhaled aerosols. They are delivered directly into the lungs where they are needed and, therefore, produce fewer side effects on other parts of the body. The medications are absorbed quickly, generally reaching their peak effect within 15 to 30 minutes, often faster than medications taken by mouth.

Inhaled aerosol treatments can be performed with a pressurized Metered Dose Delivery (MDD) device, often called a **M**etered **D**ose **I**nhaler **(MDI).** A **S**mall **V**olume **N**ebulizer **(SVN)** can be used in conjunction with a small electrical "medical" air compressor or with a compressed gas tank of oxygen or air.

Many **types of medications** can be delivered by aerosol treatments:

- *Wetting agents* like water or saline solution
- *Bronchodilators*—bronchodilators open up or dilate bronchial airways by relaxing smooth muscles that are in spasm or by controlling and keeping them open after the spasm is reversed
- *Steroids* reduce irritation, inflammation, swelling, and mucus production within the airways
- *Mucolytics* thin secretions, making it easier to clear the airways of mucus
- *Antibiotic* and *antiviral* medications work at killing infectious "bugs"

It is important to take all medications in the proper dose and **SEQUENCE,** so that you can get the maximum benefit from each one.

Metered Dose Inhaler

A metered dose inhaler (MDI) is a very simple, easy-to-handle, and convenient method of inhaling medications. An MDI, often called a "puffer," consists of a delivery device with a small container that can be filled with a variety of medicines, chiefly bronchodilators or steroids (see Chapter 4), and a mouthpiece for dispensing the drug. The advantage of this type of aerosol therapy is its direct delivery, quick action, portability, safety, and minimal care,

INSTRUCTIONS FOR METERED DOSE INHALER

1. Assemble metered dose inhaler for use. Shake well.
2. Exhale through pursed lips to a comfortable level (see Chapter 6).
3. Place the open end of the mouthpiece into your open mouth past the front teeth, as shown in the figure.

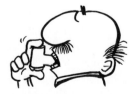

4. Do not close your lips—this allows more air to be inhaled through the mouth to aid in carrying the medication deeper into your lungs.

5. As you start taking a slow deep breath, press down firmly one time on the cartridge to release the medication.

6. Hold your breath a few seconds to allow the medication to settle on the surface of your airways. (This will prevent you from exhaling the medication and will aid in obtaining relief.)

7. Exhale slowly, using pursed lips.

8. Repeat only as prescribed; rest a minute or so before taking additional puffs, if prescribed.

9. Keep the MDI clean and free from dirt and lint by placing it in a clean plastic bag.

10. Wash and disinfect the plastic mouthpiece dispenser regularly (at least weekly).

11. Date MDI cartridges when you begin using them. Check the amount of medication in your MDI, using the "float test" so that you may obtain refills ahead of time. An easy way to estimate how much medication is left 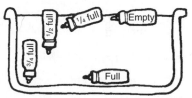 inside is to place the cartridge in a container of water and observe its position as it floats.

Note: Do not overuse. Use only as directed by your doctor.

Spacers and Extenders

Spacers and extenders are chambers placed between you and your metered dose inhaler. They allow the medication to be released first into the chamber before you inhale it. The primary advantage is to simplify the *timing* of medication release, which is so important with use of the metered dose inhalers. Spacers and extenders may also help those who experience coughing spasms when using an inhaler. In addition, they help to deliver more of the medication into the lungs and less into the mouth and throat. If your physician prescribes a spacer or extender for you, make sure that you receive instructions for use, replacement, and cleaning of the device.

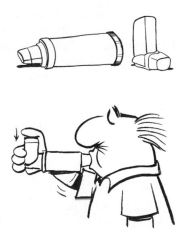

Small Volume "Wet" Nebulizers and Ultrasonic Nebulizers

A small volume "wet" nebulizer (SVN) is a medication delivery device designed to use liquid medications and sterile water or salt solutions. The solution is lifted and broken up by an airflow into a fine aerosol mist that can be inhaled.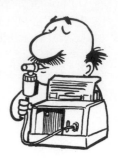

There are no clear-cut criteria for using nebulizer therapy versus metered dose inhalers for delivery of medications. Nebulizer technology came before metered dose inhalers. Both can effectively deliver inhaled aerosolized medications. SVN aerosol therapy is effective at delivering topical wetting agents.

Small volume and ultrasonic "wet" nebulizers are slightly more complicated to use than metered dose therapy. There are more parts to clean properly, disinfect, and completely air dry to minimize the potential for contamination and infection. Small volume nebulizer therapy is not as portable or as convenient as metered dose therapy, but it may have a place in the available treatment options for some patients.

AFTER YOUR TREATMENT

After each treatment, disassemble and rinse the nebulizer and mouthpiece. Shake off the excess water and place these parts on a clean paper towel. Cover with another paper towel until your next treatment.

After the last treatment of the day, follow your doctor's instructions for cleaning and disinfecting the equipment.

CARE AND CLEANING OF YOUR RESPIRATORY EQUIPMENT

You must take proper care of all equipment that delivers mists or medications into your lungs. If your equipment becomes contaminated with bacteria, even your own bacteria, you can infect yourself and put an extra strain on your lungs and heart. Be sure you clearly understand what equipment parts need to be washed and disinfected. Ask your doctor, therapist, or equipment rental company to recommend an effective technique and disinfecting agent. (We recommend daily cleaning for any mist-producing equipment.)

The following instructions offer a simple approach that is used frequently.

Supplies Needed

- Liquid detergent (such as dishwashing liquid)
- White vinegar or commercially available disinfectant
- Soft brush

- Two basins (do not use sink)
    1. Basin 1 should contain detergent water (discard daily).
    2. Basin 2 should hold one part vinegar to one part water (discard every other day; cover between use). If other disinfectants are used, they should be mixed and discarded according to the manufacturer's instructions.

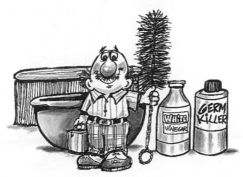

The Routine for Cleaning

1. Remove all washable parts of equipment and disassemble.
2. Wash in warm water with detergent (basin 1). Scrub all parts gently with brush. Cleaning removes medication residues, secretions, or any foreign materials.
3. Rinse thoroughly under running tap water.
4. Soak equipment in disinfecting solution (basin 2) for a minimum of 30 minutes if using vinegar or according to manufacturer's instructions if using another disinfectant (to kill bacteria). Be sure hollow parts are filled with solution and equipment is completely submerged.
5. Rinse completely under hot tap water; be careful not to let your equipment touch the sink.
6. Air-dry your equipment as follows:
    a. Shake or swing excess water out of tubing and hard-to-dry areas of accessories.
    b. Hang tubing to allow it to drip completely dry*
    c. Place all other pieces of equipment on clean paper towels and cover with clean paper towels.

---

*If you choose not to clean the nebulizer tubing, replace it often, whenever the tubing becomes hard to pinch (less pliable) or sticky when touched and when discoloration occurs.

Remember

1. Discard detergent solution (basin 1) daily.
2. Vinegar solution (basin 2) should be covered and can be kept for 2 days, but no longer. Store in a clean area.
3. Wipe down all surfaces of the machine with a clean damp cloth daily. Then cover and store the machine in a clean area between treatments.

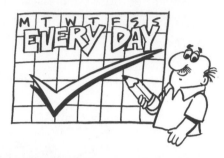

4. Use the scrub brush and basins only for cleaning *this equipment*.
5. Store dry tubing and accessories in new sealed plastic bags.
6. Have two complete sets of washable equipment so you always have a clean, dry setup available for use the following day.
7. Hair dryers or blowers are not to be used to dry equipment.

    All equipment must be washed as stated every 24 hours!

How to Prepare Sterilized Water or Normal Saline Solution for Home Use

Here are instructions for making your own solutions for inhalation. It may be less expensive for you to prepare them than to buy them. However, it may be more convenient to purchase prepared normal saline solution (a mild salt solution) to use with your medication. Remember that bacteria can grow in your solutions unless you are extremely careful. Please follow these instructions exactly as they are written.

1. You need a jar with a lid that fits snugly. A small jam jar or juice bottle will do.
2. Thoroughly wash this jar and its lid in detergent; rinse.
3. Place the jar and its lid in a clean pan and fill with tap water so that the jar is completely submerged. Place a lid on the pan and gently boil the jar for 15 minutes to sterilize it.
4. After you have boiled the jar, pour the tap water out of the pan. (Use the pan lid to prevent the sterilized jar from falling out.)
5. After the jar and lid have cooled, remove them from the pan. Place them upright on a clean counter. Do not let anything "unsterile" touch the insides of the jar or lid. Do not dry them with a towel or place them upside down to drain.
6. Resterilize the jar and lid at least once each week.

7. Pour distilled water (twice the desired amount) into the clean pan used to boil the jar. If preparing normal saline solution (salt water), add ¼ teaspoon of salt to every 2 cups of distilled water.

8. Boil gently for 15 minutes. You will have about half the water you started with. Let the water cool and then pour it into the "sterile" jar; cover it with the "sterile" lid.

9. Store this in the refrigerator. Discard any unused solutions at least once a week.

10. To remove any solution from the jar, pour directly into your nebulizer. Never place an "unsterilized" eyedropper, teaspoon, or other measuring device into the solution in the jar. Do not pour any extra solution back into the jar once it has been removed—discard it.

Saline or diluent solutions may be purchased from pharmacies in cans without a prescription or in prepackaged vials that require a prescription. These may be more expensive, but they are convenient and provide accurately measured doses.

6

The Art of Better Breathing and Coughing

CORRECT BREATHING TECHNIQUES AND EXERCISES

Most people take breathing for granted until something causes them to have difficulty getting air into or out of their lungs. Many people breathe inefficiently, often as the result of early posture training. This causes them to work harder than they need to with every breath they take. Breathing exercises can be done by anyone to help improve breathing efficiency and decrease the work of breathing.

In obstructive lung diseases like COPD, airways can collapse as you exhale and trap stale air in the alveoli/air sacs. When this happens, your lungs become overfilled with stale air and there isn't enough room for you to breathe in fresh air. Correct breathing techniques can increase breathing efficiency, which helps minimize the trapped air and the uncomfortable feelings of shortness of breath.

Pursed Lips Breathing

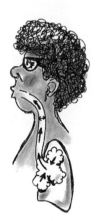

The pursed lips breathing technique provides a resistance to exhaled air at the mouth and maintains a higher pressure in the airways. This keeps the airways open longer so that you can lift and squeeze with your abdominal muscles and push more air out. This makes room for a fresh breath of oxygenated air and reduces your shortness of breath. Pursed lips breathing can be done by pursing or puckering your lips into a whistling or kissing position, then blowing slowly and gently. It can also be done by gently placing your tongue flat against the roof of your mouth, with your lips barely open, while exhaling slowly past your tongue to remove stale trapped air from your lungs.

1. Take a comfortable breath in through your nose with your mouth closed.
2. Exhale slowly and gently through your mouth with your lips pursed.

Belly Breathing

Belly breathing exercises recruit, reactivate and strengthen the abdominal/ belly muscles and assist the action of the diaphragm. Normally the diaphragm does about 80% of the work of breathing. In patients with COPD, or in normal persons with well-intentioned posture training, the diaphragm can be pushed down and/or become less active. Then the muscles of the upper chest and neck take over and are used more for breathing. These muscles are less efficient and require more oxygen to do the diaphragm's job. To locate your diaphragm, place your flat hand on your abdomen just below your breastbone—then sniff. You can feel your diaphragm move with your belly.

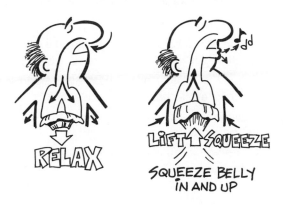

RELAX

LIFT SQUEEZE

SQUEEZE BELLY
IN AND UP

To do belly breathing, you *actively* contract your chest and abdominal muscles as you exhale. Squeeze inward and upward, lifting and compressing your abdominal ("belly") contents against your diaphragm. This squeezes your lungs to get the stale air out. Don't force the air out to the point of discomfort. Relax the belly and chest muscles to inhale.

Each person will have his or her own comfortable length of time to exhale. To establish *your* exhalation time, count during several comfortable exhalations. Don't force air out to the point of discomfort. The ratio of inhalation time to exhalation time (I:E ratio) often differs from one person to another and with the condition of the lungs. The I:E ratio for normal lungs is, generally, about 1:1.5; that is, you exhale 1½ times as long as you inhale. For persons with COPD, it takes longer to exhale so that exhalation is often twice or more longer than inhalation. For example, If you have COPD, think to yourself, "in 2" then "out 2, 3, 4" as you slowly exhale, tightening inward and upward with your belly muscles to squeeze the trapped air out. You may need to spend even *more* time getting the stale air out. Relax your chest and belly muscles to take in the next breath of fresh air. For those with restrictive lung diseases, shorter and quicker breaths (e.g., I:E ratio of 1:1) seem to work best. It all takes practice.

Pursed lips and belly breathing are the basic techniques used with all breathing exercises, physical exertion, or activities. They should be used whenever you do work, or if your breathing *becomes* work. Remember to "whistle when you work." Whenever you become short of breath, pursed lips breathing should be practiced along with correct and comfortable belly breathing. Learn these first and learn them well.

 Exercise CORRECT BREATHING TECHNIQUES— COORDINATING PURSED LIPS AND BELLY BREATHING

Assume a comfortable position.

1 Place one hand in the center of your abdomen at the base of your breastbone—this hand will detect the movement of your belly and diaphragm.

2 Place your other hand on your upper chest—this hand will detect any movement of your chest and accessory muscles.

3 Exhale slowly through pursed lips while pulling your abdominal muscles inward, squeezing them upward (Figures A and B).

4 Inhale through your nose—your abdomen should drop downward and expand outward (Figures C and D). The hand on the belly should feel the most movement.

5 Rest.

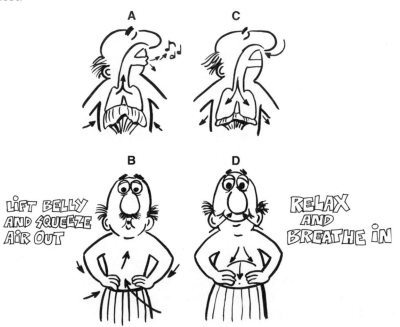

Practice combining this exercise as part of your home exercise program.

It is necessary to practice often in order to strengthen and coordinate your muscles. Set aside several (three to five) times throughout the day to practice. Be sure to rest after five deep breaths, or you may overbreathe and become lightheaded. Concentrate on making each breath slow and deep. Pursed lips with belly breathing should always be used first to clear out the stale air when you practice *correct breathing*.

Correct breathing (pursed lips/belly breathing) can become your normal breathing pattern if practiced faithfully; this will result in less shortness of breath. Correct pursed lips/belly breathing should be used during exercise and during strenuous activities, as well as during episodes of shortness of breath. Master these techniques before going on to other exercises.

Controlled Coughing Technique

Coughing is the natural way of removing foreign substances from the airways and lungs. Patients with chronic lung disease often produce an excess of mucus. Excess mucus must be removed to maintain open airways and allow you to move air in and out of your lungs effectively. If the excess mucus is not removed, shortness of breath can worsen. Retained mucus can also contribute to the risk of infection. In addition, the mucus irritates nerve endings in the tracheobronchial tree and can cause frequent, involuntary coughing, resulting in bronchial muscle spasms and fatigue. To conserve energy and oxygen, practice and master the method of controlled coughing.

Step 1—Hold a tissue in front of your mouth and nose to control aerosol droplets.

Step 2—At the end of a comfortable pursed lips exhalation, take a slow deep breath, using correct breathing. Slowly build up a volume of air behind the mucus to help to propel it toward the mouth.

Step 3—Hold the deep breath and increase pressure for several seconds.

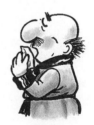

Right

Step 4—Make two short, staccato coughs with your mouth slightly open. The first cough loosens the mucus, and the second cough moves it upward to be cleared.

Step 5—Pause.

Step 6—Inhale by sniffing gently or make a few short, rapid exhalations until you can take in another slow correct breath. Taking in a big fast breath after coughing may cause you to cough again or may draw the mucus back into the lungs.

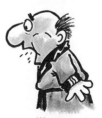

Wrong

Step 7—Rest.

Breathing humidified air and taking a drink of water before coughing can be helpful. It may also help to take your inhaled medications before coughing. Coughing is easier when you are in a sitting position with your head slightly forward. Controlled, effective coughing should make a hollow sound.

COUGHING STEPS IN BRIEF

1. Cover your mouth and nose with a tissue.
2. Breathe in through your nose, slowly and deeply.
3. Hold your breath and increase chest/abdominal pressure.
4. Make two short, staccato coughs.
5. Pause.
6. Inhale by sniffing slowly and gently or puff/pant to get control, if needed.
7. Rest.

If you need to cough again, repeat the procedure step by step. Control your cough; don't let it control *you*.

More ways of clearing mucus from your airways are covered in detail in Chapter 8 ("Cleaning Out Your Tubes: Bronchial Hygiene").

7

Day In, Day Out: Your Daily Activities

Our bodies are the most amazing and complicated pieces of equipment that we will ever use. The body's efficiency depends on our ability to recognize and use its superb physical design and natural functions. The use of proper body mechanics and efficient breathing techniques while going about your daily routine will enable you to do more with less shortness of breath, fatigue, and risk of injury.

Remember to pace your exertion and activities within comfortable, efficient breathing patterns. Whistle when you work, doing most of the exertion while you exhale. Another hint will help you work with your body's natural movements: **inhale as you expand your chest, and exhale when you compress your chest and/or abdomen.** Pace your work to your comfortable, controlled breathing capacity. If you feel like taking a couple of breaths between the work, do so—then continue as described. It is not necessary to do work on every exhalation. Just be sure to keep the air moving.

RULES FOR COORDINATING CORRECT BREATHING WITH EXERTION

1. Begin all exertion, exercises, and work with correct breathing techniques (CBT), with emphasis on a pursed lip/belly breathing exhalation to clear stale air from the lungs.

2. Take a comfortably deep breath before doing any work (especially something strenuous).

3. Exhale during the exertion part of any work. The only exception is to inhale when expanding the chest and exhale when compressing the chest or abdomen.

4. If you have COPD (obstructive lung disease), breathe out at least twice as long as you breathe in (i.e., inhale to the count of 2, exhale to the count of 4). If you have restrictive lung disease, you may be more comfortable if your inhalation and exhalation are about equal (i.e., in to the count of 2, then out to the count of 2). (See Chapter 6 for specific breathing instructions.)

5. If your oxygen prescription includes use with exertion, it includes everyday activities like showering, grooming, and moving about, as well as exercise. You and your physician will decide what is best for you.

REDEVELOPING GOOD POSTURE

Maintaining a well-balanced carriage is as essential to habitual good breathing as using your respiratory and abdominal muscles. Good balance and posture also help to relax the muscles of the shoulders, neck, and upper chest. The following basic points should be considered and practiced:

1. Stand comfortably straight and tall, not "tin soldier" rigid. Stand with at least half your body weight carried forward over the front of the feet so that the toes are pressed onto the ground.

2. Practice rocking forward, onto your toes, until the heels have to come off the ground—then backward until the toes do. Settle between these two extremes. The weight should be evenly divided between the front of the foot and the heel. In most cases it is necessary to accentuate the forward shifting of your weight.

3. Stand sideways in front of a long mirror and note the following:
   a. Is your head pushing forward? Correct this by stretching upward and tucking your chin in while pressing your head backward.
   b. Do your shoulders hunch forward or upward? Bring your shoulder blades down and back.
   c. Is your seat sticking out? Tuck in the seat muscles and relax your shoulders and upper chest.

4. When sitting in a chair, sit well back in the seat and support your legs with feet flat on the floor (never dangle them). Support your arms on armrests or a table or place them on your lap.

5. Pelvic tilt. To do a pelvic tilt exercise:
   a. Stand with your back against the wall, as described above. You can also do this pelvic tilt exercise while sitting or while lying on your back with your knees bent and feet flat on the floor or bed.
   b. While exhaling, contract the abdominal muscles slowly and roll your hips so that your back is flat against the wall, floor, or bed.
   c. Relax your muscles and rest.

Practice Posture Work Against a Wall for About 5 Minutes at a Time

Assume the following position:

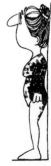

1. With your back against the wall, place feet several inches apart and a few inches away from the wall.

2. Hold head high.

3. Tuck chin in.

4. Relax shoulders.

5. Tuck hips under in a pelvic tilt.

6. Slightly flex knees.

When you feel that you can hold the position properly, try standing away from the wall in the proper postural position, and then attempt to walk in this position.

You will notice that the trunk stays quite rigid when you are standing but that the legs (hips and knees) bend more when you are walking. Try to relax your muscles as much as possible. Check to see whether you have retained the proper position by backing up to the wall during your walking practice. Do not stiffen up when trying to maintain a proper posture. Only by being relaxed can you benefit from this exercise.

BODY MECHANICS

The joints and bones in your body are like the parts of a machine and will wear out if they are strained too much or incorrectly. Also, advancing age and long-term use of medicines such as steroids may make bones brittle. Proper body mechanics are essential to help your body function effectively.

Proper Body Mechanics Tips

- It is important that your breathing and your body movements are smooth and steady, never jerky, sudden, or strained.

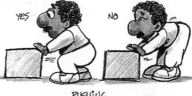

YES NO

PUSHING

- Do not lift, push, or pull when your back is twisted or bent. Use your feet to turn around and lift by bending and straightening your knees. When you lift an object, it should be held as close to your body as possible.
- Avoid carrying heavy items in your arms; instead, use a rolling cart for moving groceries, laundry, tools, and equipment.

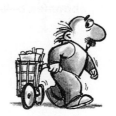

- Work at the proper height so you can avoid sustained back bending or having to lift your arms too high. Proper work height is generally a couple of inches below your elbows, for both the standing and sitting positions.

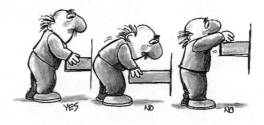

YES NO NO

- Never sit in a chair that's too low or too high; have your back, feet, and arms well supported. You will generally feel more comfortable sitting erect or even leaning slightly forward.

Standing Up from a Chair

1. Do a CBT cycle to cleanse your lungs.
2. Take a deep breath by using your belly while you are relaxed.
3. While breathing out through pursed lips, move forward on the chair. Take another breath in, then rise straight up to your feet. "Whistle while you work."

Going Up a Flight of Stairs or Walking Up a Hill

1. Do a correct breathing cycle to cleanse your lungs.
2. While standing relaxed, before you start to climb, take a slow, deep breath by using correct breathing. While exhaling through pursed lips and using belly breathing, climb two or three stairs or take two or three steps up the incline. Count your paced breathing, "Out 2, 3, 4" as you step up one step per count; hesitate while breathing "In 2."
3. Stop and rest, relaxing your chest and belly, while breathing in again.
4. If you feel short of breath at this point, rest for a while, taking as many breaths as needed to feel comfortable again. When you are ready, continue in the manner just described.

Bending

Bending to tie shoes, put on socks, or pick up fallen treasures requires compressing the abdomen/belly against the diaphragm and chest. Work **with** your body; **exhale through pursed lips whenever you bend, compressing the abdomen/belly and chest.**

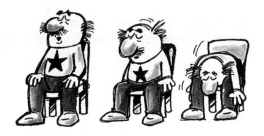

Lifting Loads

Do CBT before beginning to do work. Before lifting, straighten the spine by doing a pelvic tilt to reduce low back stress. Take a deep breath while you are relaxed. Bend at the knees and hips, not at the waist. Exhale through pursed lips, using belly breathing; when lifting, hold the load close to your body and place the load where you wish.

REMEMBER TO

1. Inhale as you expand your chest.
2. Exhale through pursed lips when you compress your chest or diaphragm.
3. Whistle as you do the exertion part of the work.

Many people with chronic lung disease regard all arm movements, especially movements from the shoulders, as difficult and tiresome. The following examples show how to coordinate proper breathing with these movements.

Pushing a Broom, Vacuum Cleaner, or Lawn Mower

Do CBT to cleanse the lungs before beginning work. Relax and take a deep breath before you start to push anything. Maintaining a relaxed straight posture, push objects while exhaling with pursed lips and using belly breathing. Stop and rest while inhaling. Continue coordinating breathing with pushing and pulling objects.

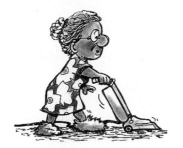 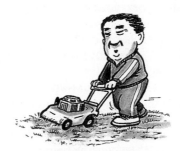

Raising the Arms to Reach or Do Work At or Above Shoulder Level

Do CBT to cleanse the lungs before beginning work. Relax and take a deep breath as you lift your arms to shoulder level, expanding your chest and reaching for the intended goal. Exhale as you exert yourself or retrieve the object and then lower your arms.

Shaving and Combing Hair

Do CBT to cleanse your lungs before beginning work. Relax and take a deep breath as you lift your arms and expand your chest. While exhaling, shave or comb two or three strokes. Lower your arms and rest before you run out of air. Your arms should be back in a resting position at the end of that comfortable exhalation. Do CBT, if necessary, between activities. Remember that you do not need to work during each exhalation.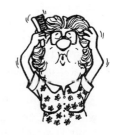

Some Additional Examples of When You Might Use This Breathing Technique

Personal hygiene—showering, brushing teeth, dressing

Household tasks—bed making, window washing, mopping, moving furniture, meal preparation and clean up

Exercises—breathing exercises, walking, bicycle riding, swimming, body improvement exercises, relaxation exercises, bronchial hygiene

Hobbies—crafts, singing, golfing, bowling, dancing

Garden work—digging, planting, weeding, pruning, raking

SOME EXAMPLES OF ENERGY SAVING TECHNIQUES

Saving your energy can be important in order to complete your necessary daily chores. Often this can be accomplished by slight changes in the way you prioritize or perform these tasks.

- Plan your daily chores in advance, so that you won't feel rushed or have to push beyond your limitations.
- Decide which jobs are absolutely necessary and which are desirable to make your home comfortable and attractive.
- Adopt a cooperative work-sharing attitude within your family. Assign tasks and responsibilities.
- Pace all work to your own breathing comfort and speed.
- Distribute tedious tasks throughout the week.
- Do the tasks requiring the most exertion when you have the most energy. For example, if mornings are difficult, take your shower and set the breakfast table the evening before.
- Alternate easy and difficult activities, and take rest periods between activities to prevent becoming overfatigued.
- Save 50% of your energy: sit down to do your work. Use a stool at the kitchen counter, at the work bench, or in the shower.
- Drain dishes; let them air dry instead of towel drying.
- Prepare food for two or more meals at one cooking session. Refrigerate or freeze individual-sized meals for another time.
- Minimize clutter in storage areas, cupboards, closets, wardrobes, and tool sheds so that you can easily find and reach what you need.
- Avoid ironing clothes by using easy-care, no-iron fabrics.
- Straighten up rooms as you go along. A good rule for you and household members/guests is "never leave a room empty-handed."
- Vacuuming may leave fine dust in the air. Lightly misting the bag will reduce the number of escaping particles. To minimize breathing in these particles, try using a moist handkerchief in front of your mouth and nose while vacuuming; open windows and let the room air out for at least an hour. Use only disposable vacuum bags and change them often.

- When making your bed, start at the head and progress down one side toward and across the foot, tucking in and smoothing as you go. Then proceed up the other side. Casters make moving the bed easier. It is more convenient if only the head of the bed is against the wall. Use an electric blanket. They are lightweight, easy to lift, and don't weigh heavily on your body at night.

SOME TIPS FOR DAILY SELF-CARE

Your hygiene and grooming can be some of the more strenuous and exerting activities you have to do in a day. Sit while washing, showering, dressing, grooming, and applying makeup to conserve 50% of your energy!

- A short, easy-to-maintain haircut requires less work, energy, and breath.
- Try an electric toothbrush if brushing is a chore.
- If steam in the shower bothers you, try turning on the cold water first and then slowly adding the hot. Leave bathroom windows and doors open as much as possible to increase airflow and decrease steam buildup. Consider using a fan. The air does not necessarily have to be fresh for you to breathe comfortably, as long as it circulates.
- Be sure to use your oxygen in the shower or bath if it has been prescribed for use with activity. The portable tank, with extra-long tubing, can be set just outside the shower or tub.
- If you feel short of breath under an overhead shower or when splashing water on your face, use a washcloth, and install a hand shower to control the direction and force of the water flow.
- To dry after bathing or showering, try wrapping yourself in a lightweight terry cloth robe. Its absorbent qualities will dry you automatically. Rubbing yourself dry after a bath can be very tiring.
- Grab bars and no-slip strips in the tub or shower will help you keep your balance.
- Avoid scented soaps, colognes, and other grooming products if you find they bother your breathing.
- Keep your movements small and close to your body. You don't need to reach the ceiling to wash under your arms. To scrub hard-to-reach areas, like feet or back, use long-handled tools or a folded towel with handles at each end and a brush or loofah sponge attached in the middle. This can be pulled diagonally back and forth to give a good scrub.

Remember to coordinate your breathing techniques with all activities.

1. Relax the accessory muscles when you inhale.
2. Use pursed lips and squeeze with the abdominal muscles and belly while you exhale.
3. Exhale at least twice as long as you inhale.
4. Begin all activities with CBT, starting with an exhalation to cleanse the lungs of trapped, stale air.
5. Inhale when expanding the chest and lungs.
6. Exhale, using belly breathing, when compressing the chest and/or abdomen.

8
Cleaning Out Your Tubes: Bronchial Hygiene

The respiratory system is constantly exposed to and working to overcome bombardment by all of the pollutants, fumes, irritants, and infectious materials that are in the air we breathe. Our bodies normally produce a thin layer of mucous secretions to help moisten and protect our lungs from these atmospheric invaders. The special hairlike cilia are working to keep the mucus moving upward, to be swallowed or coughed up.

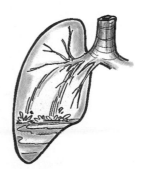

Many people with chronic lung diseases have extra secretions in their bronchial tubes. Everyone gets an acute respiratory infection now and then, which can cause an increase in secretions. When secretions are excessive (more than 1½ to 2 tablespoons in a day), they can cause problems. Secretions tend to pool in the lower parts of the lungs because of gravity. This not only makes it more difficult to breathe but also may interfere with getting oxygen into the blood. These secretions are also a perfect place for bacteria to grow and multiply and cause lung infections. By removing these secretions, you will be able to breathe more easily, reduce or prevent infections, and generally feel better.

Secretions tend to pool in the bottom of your lungs because you spend most of your time in the upright position. To get secretions to a point where you can cough them up more easily, you need to use mucus-clearing bronchial hygiene techniques. To assess and evaluate your individual and specific need for one or more of these techniques, discuss this with your doctor, respiratory therapist, or rehabilitation specialist. Some techniques and devices will require a prescription.

Bronchial hygiene techniques may include any or all of the following. Be sure you have received proper instruction (and a prescription, if needed) before beginning these.

- Correct breathing techniques (pursed lips exhalation with belly breathing) with the use of controlled cough or huff cough techniques
- Positive expiratory pressure (PEP)—used with pursed lips breathing and by the TheraPEP device
- Autogenic drainage (AD)
- Flutter valve
- Bronchial drainage (BD)

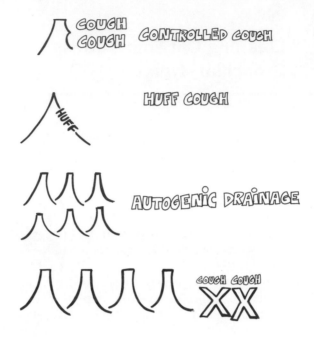

- Chest physiotherapy (CPT)—percussion or vibration provided manually or with a mechanical device
- Exercise

STEPS TO FOLLOW FOR EFFECTIVE BRONCHIAL HYGIENE

Step 1—**CONDITION airways and secretions: medicate, humidify, and liquefy**
- Take prescribed medications to dilate your airways before you begin bronchial hygiene. Oral bronchodilator medicine should ideally be taken at least 45 minutes beforehand. Inhaled bronchodilator medicines should be taken *at least* 10 minutes before you do bronchial hygiene.
- Drink a minimum of 1½ to 2 quarts of caffeine-free or nonalcoholic liquids daily. Adequate fluid intake is necessary to keep mucus thin.
- Breathing highly humidified air, from any safe source, can help to thin secretions.

Step 2—**INFLATE the lungs and MOBILIZE secretions**
Use breathing and coughing techniques, medical devices, gravity, percussion, and vibration. Talk with your doctor, rehabilitation specialist, or respiratory therapist for instruction in these techniques.
- **Breathing exercises** are very important. Pursed lips and belly breathing should be done throughout the bronchial hygiene period.

- **Pursed lips breathing** is one way of exerting back pressure in the airways. It is one method of **positive expiratory pressure** (PEP). PEP helps to widen your airways so secretions can be mobilized and cleared more easily and to minimize shortness of breath while clearing secretions. The **TheraPEP** device uses this technology but requires a prescription.
- Forced exhalations, or **autogenic drainage** in conjunction with "huff" coughing, are breathing techniques used specifically to help loosen and mobilize secretions. Autogenic drainage is simply breathing repetitively at different, increasing depths and then performing breath holding and forced exhalations ending in a controlled or huff 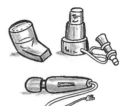 cough. (See illustration on p. 56.) The specific technique for AD can be taught to you by your respiratory therapist or pulmonary rehabilitation specialist.
- **Flutter**—The flutter device is a small pipe engineered with an internal cone and a heavy steel ball bearing. Exhaled airflow causes the steel ball to lift and fall, causing vibrations in the airflow and internally within the airways. These oscillations and pressure changes mobilize and thin bronchial secretions. The flutter device requires a prescription.
- **Bronchial drainage/postural drainage** (PD) uses gravity to move secretions from small airways into larger airways for easier clearance. Gravity can be an important consideration in the draining of secretions. Check with your doctor before doing gravity positioning. If head-lower-than-hips positions are needed, your doctor, therapist, or nurse will need to prescribe them and discuss the cautions regarding getting into a head-down position. The positions in the figures show gravity drainage positions. Stay in each position (1 through 4) for 5 to 15 minutes.

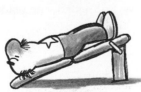

1. Both lower lobes
   (on back—pillow under knee)

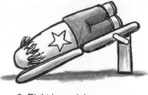

2. Right lower lobe
   (straight up on left side)

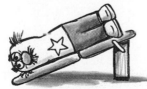

3. Left lower lobe
   (straight up on right side)

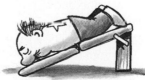

4. Both lower lobes
   (lie on stomach)

- Manual and mechanical **percussion and vibration** are additional methods of loosening and moving secretions. Percussion, or clapping with a cupped hand on the chest wall, helps to move secretions into the larger airways. Percussion should be done only on the rib cage and not over the spinal column, breastbone, or soft tissues. Percussion may be prescribed for at least 1 minute in each position. Vibration is another means of moving secretions. Your rib cage can be vibrated by another person or by a mechanical device. Vibration should follow percussion and is done for an additional minute only when you are exhaling. Your skin should be covered with clothing or a towel during percussion and vibration. Your doctor or therapist should instruct you in these procedures.
- **Exercise** is another way of increasing pressure and airflow changes in the bronchial tubes and of mobilizing secretions. As you breathe more deeply and rapidly, during exercise—or even for an hour or so after exercise—you may find that you have an increased ability to cough up mucus.

Step 3—**COUGH and CLEAR secretions**
- **Controlled** and **huff coughing** have been shown to effectively loosen and clear secretions. These coughing techniques can be used alone or in conjunction with any of the other bronchial hygiene techniques. Be sure to sit upright before using any coughing technique.

Step 4—**REST**

BASIC POINTS

- Bronchial hygiene is best done first thing in the morning (1 hour before or 2 hours after eating) and in the evening (same time frame around eating and at least 1 hour before bedtime).
- Do bronchial hygiene at least once or twice daily. Increase the number of treatments to three or four if your secretions change color or increase in amount or when you have a cold.
- When you feel least like doing your bronchial hygiene technique, you probably need it the most.
- If you use supplemental oxygen, be sure to use it while doing your bronchial hygiene.
- If postural/bronchial drainage is prescribed, it is important to tilt the chest area 10 to 20 degrees below the horizontal level. This can be accomplished by using one of the following suggested methods:
  A slant board
  Couch pillows placed on the floor
  Firm pillows propped under your hips in bed
- Cough after each position, but only when you are sitting upright. Use the controlled coughing techniques.
- Rest after coughing.

REMEMBER THESE FOUR KEY STEPS:

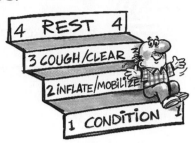

1. **CONDITION** airways and secretions.
2. **INFLATE** lungs and **MOBILIZE** secretions.
3. **COUGH** and **CLEAR.**
4. **REST.**

9

Exercise to Better Health

WHERE TO BEGIN

Good physical condition is an objective that every-one should seek, including the person with chronic lung disease. Persons with chronic lung disease frequently avoid physical activity because of the limitations imposed by shortness of breath. In addition, friends, family, or physicians may have encouraged them not to exert themselves, assuming that doing so might be harmful. Inactivity works against you. Sitting or lying around deconditions the body and makes your muscles less strong and less efficient.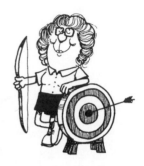
This, in turn, makes doing even the simplest daily activities more difficult with regard to both energy and breathing. This deconditioning effect can be reversed by a regular exercise program.

With progressive exercise, muscles become stronger and more resistant to fatigue. With practice and training, you learn to perform tasks more efficiently; that is, you need less oxygen for the same amount of work. Thus you may have more "energy" to accomplish the tasks you perform each day, and you may do these tasks with less shortness of breath.

The techniques described in this chapter will not help the lungs themselves but will improve your entire physical condition. The reconditioning of muscles should be undertaken with great care, since suddenly starting to exercise may be unsafe. Check with your physician before beginning an exercise program. Careful evaluation of the type and extent of your pulmonary limitations is essential before establishing a physical conditioning program.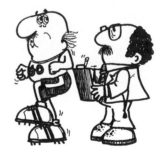

Each part of your physical conditioning program should be checked for safety before you attempt it. For example, walking too fast or too far may put excessive strain on your lungs or heart. Or certain physical activities may cause your blood oxygen level to fall too low, requiring supplemental oxygen during exercise. Do not attempt to construct your own program. Your doctor and other health care professionals can guide you within safe limits. These limits can be established by appropriate testing. The program can then be tailored to your abilities. There are no simple guidelines that you can establish. For instance, becoming short of breath during a given exercise does not mean that you are overdoing it and have to stop. If it did, most athletes would stop in the middle of a race, a tennis match, or a football game. Remember to use correct breathing techniques. If you have obstructive lung disease, try to exhale twice as long as you inhale. If you have restrictive lung disease you may be more comfortable if your inhalation and exhalation are equal. Even fatigue or aching muscles do not necessarily mean you are overdoing it. It may be necessary to experience such discomforts to improve your condition. However, "no pain, no gain" is a fallacy. Let your physician set the limits based on detailed knowledge of your condition.

Whatever the exercise program designed for you, you will be responsible for mastering it. You will find that you may have to push yourself to establish a regular routine. Being short of breath creates a temptation to remain inactive, especially on the days when your shortness of breath 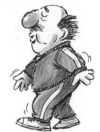 may seem worse. When planning a safe exercise schedule, remember to start slowly. Plan a progressive walking program, beginning with short distances and a slow pace. You may gradually increase the duration of your walks as your strength and endurance increase. Keep a careful record of your exercise sessions (for example, how long you walked, how fast you walked, and how you tolerated the exercise). Then you and your doctor can monitor your progress and adjust your exercise routine as necessary. Setting aside a specific time to exercise may help to establish a regular regimen. Keep a regularly scheduled exercise time on "bad breathing days" and replace your normal routine with an alternative activity that is at a lower level. Finding a companion to exercise with can make your exercise program more enjoyable and help with motivation.

SAFETY GUIDELINES

1. Check with your physician before beginning an exercise program.
2. Wear loose, comfortable clothing that does not restrict movement of your chest or abdomen.
3. Wait at least 1 hour after a meal before you exercise.
4. The best time of day to exercise depends on you, your ability to breathe, and your schedule.
5. Walk on level areas. If you encounter an incline, you will need to slow your pace.
6. Do not attempt to walk outdoors in inclement weather or during times of smog alerts. If necessary, walk inside your home or go to an enclosed shopping mall.

7. Report any adverse symptoms to your medical professional.
8. Always use oxygen if prescribed during exercise; allow 3 to 10 minutes of oxygenation time before exercise.
9. Use bronchodilators before exercise.
10. Wear supportive shoes.
11. Proper posture is important when exercising in a chair. Sit with your hip and knee joints at 90-degree angles and with your feet flat on the floor. Press your lower back firmly against the back of the chair while exercising. Do not allow an increase in the curvature of your lower back.

COMPONENTS OF YOUR EXERCISE PROGRAM
Endurance Exercise

Most persons with chronic lung disease have become inactive because of shortness of breath or fear. Deconditioned muscles require more effort than conditioned muscles to do the same amount of work. Regular exercise is the way to build your endurance.

Decide what type of exercise you would like to participate in, what you have access to, and what you enjoy. The kind of exercise that will benefit you the most depends on what you want to do. Exercise training is specific; i.e., walking exercise helps you to become a more efficient walker. If you walk for exercise, then walking to doctor appointments, social engagements, and shopping may seem easier. Other types of exercise are also beneficial— swimming, bicycling, dancing, etc. All of these are aerobic activities, exercises that require oxygen, use your large muscle groups, and can be sustained for a period of time.

Each endurance exercise session should include three phases: A **warm-up,** the **training level,** the **cool-down.**

The **warm-up** phase of your exercise program should precede stretching and endurance training. It should be 3 to 5 minutes in duration, with gradual increases of intensity to your target. The purpose of the warm-up is to prepare the body for the greater demands of exercise by increasing blood flow and oxygen to the muscles. This increase in your internal temperature improves muscle elasticity, increases flexibility of tendons and ligaments, and decreases the potential risk of injury. Beginning exercise too suddenly may cause abnormal heartbeats, constrict your airways, or possibly increase shortness of breath. Bronchodilators should be nearby and should be used before beginning exercise. Movements used in the warm-up should specifically prepare the body for movements used during the exercise component. If you are going to walk, you can do chair exercises that simulate walking or walk at a slower pace.

Duration of the aerobic phase is related to your capacity and may vary from a few minutes to an hour. The **frequency** may vary from three 5-minute sessions or two 15-minute sessions daily to one 30-minute session every day or every other day. The recommended frequency is 3 to 5 days per week.

The **cool-down** should always follow endurance training. It is necessary to safely return to your resting state. Stopping abruptly can cause dizziness and abnormal heartbeats. Gradually decrease intensity for approximately 3 to 5 minutes, thereby lowering your heart rate, preventing pooling of blood in the lower extremities, and reducing muscle soreness.

Arm-R-Size

People with lung disease often become short of breath when doing activities with their arms. This causes them to do fewer and fewer upper body activities that are important for many activities of daily living, such as washing, dressing, or grooming. This inactivity causes the arm and shoulder muscles to become weak. Upper body training can be used to regain the strength and endurance of these muscles.

Arm-R-Size is an endurance activity for your upper body. It is designed to be performed while sitting in a chair. The following is a list of some Arm-R-Size movements. You have artistic freedom in interpreting how to perform these movements. These movements can be simplified by keeping your arms below shoulder level. To get started, you can perform any five of these movements for 1 minute each. As your endurance improves, you can gradually increase the **duration** toward a goal of 15 minutes—by adding more activities or increasing the time of each one. When you reach 15 minutes of continuous exercise, you can increase the **intensity** by adding 0.5 to 1 pound of hand weights or soup cans. Use these intermittently until they can be used continuously for 15 minutes. The recommended **frequency** is 3 to 5 days per week. Remember to coordinate these exercises with pursed lip breathing.

Punching bag	Arm jog
Marching soldier	Pump the tire
Windshield wipers	Crawlstroke
Breaststroke	Play the piano
Play the drums	Pull the tug-o-war rope
Wax the car	Drive the bus
Upper cuts	Pull the weeds
Row the boat	Stir the soup in the cauldron
Reach for the stars	Swing the bat

Have fun with this and feel free to invent your own movements. Arm-R-Size can be performed any place, any time without any special equipment. It is also a good lower-level activity to perform on days when you have more symptoms.

STRETCHING FOR FLEXIBILITY

Stretching is necessary to increase and maintain adequate range of motion in your joints. Flexibility can ease the performance of daily activities, decrease risk of injury, and improve mobility. Flexibility exercises should stretch the major muscle groups: neck, shoulder, back, chest, arms, hips, legs, and calves. The best time to stretch is after you have warmed up or after endurance training. Warming up first helps to increase circulation and body temperature. Stretching muscles that have not been warmed up may cause injury and impede increased flexibility.

Stretch slowly and smoothly to the point of mild discomfort. Never bounce or stretch to a point that causes pain. Optimally hold each stretch for 10 to 30 seconds, or as long as it feels comfortable. Perform two to three repetitions of each exercise 2 to 5 days per week. Stretching is also a good lower-level activity to perform on days when you have more symptoms.

The shoulder and neck muscles are considered accessory breathing muscles and are not normally involved in the work of quiet breathing. Some persons with chronic lung disease tend to breathe shallowly, using their upper chest muscles because of decreased mobility of the rib cage and flattening of the diaphragm. To breathe properly, you must relax your shoulder and neck muscles. The following exercises can be done any time during the day when you feel tension in the shoulder and neck area. To increase flexibility, they should be done as part of your stretching routine.

 Exercise HEAD CIRCLING

1 Roll your head slowly from side to side in a forward semicircle.

2 Repeat a couple of times.

3 *Do not* arch your neck by rolling your head back.

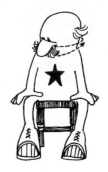

Exercise SHOULDER SHRUGGING

1 Stand or sit with feet slightly apart and arms relaxed.
2 Shrug your shoulders up toward your ears and hold.
3 Relax and repeat.

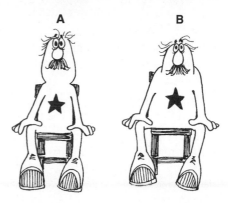

 Exercise ELBOW CIRCLING

1 Sit or stand with hands on shoulders.
2 Circle the elbows forward, up, back, and downward. Do 2 to 10 circles.

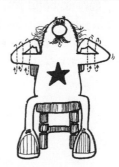

 Exercise CIRCLING OF SHOULDERS WITH HANGING ARMS

1 Sit or stand with arms relaxed.
2 Circle both shoulders backward 10 times.
3 Circle both shoulders forward 10 times.

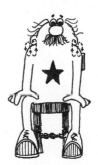

Exercise OVER-THE-HEAD SHOULDER STRETCH

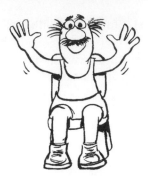

1 Sit and press your lower back firmly against the back of the chair.

2 Pretend you are holding a stick. Keep both arms outstretched 3 feet apart. Do not lock your elbows.

3 Slowly raise your extended arms above your head to the point where the tops of your shoulders feel tight.

4 Return to starting position.

 Exercise UNDERNEATH SHOULDER STRETCH

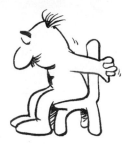

1 Sit and bend your head and chest forward slightly.

2 Reach your arms behind your back, clasp your hands together, and lift slowly.

3 Return to starting position.

 Exercise SIDE BENDING

1 Sit up straight with feet apart.

2 Bend your trunk to the side.

3 Return to starting position.

A   B

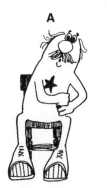
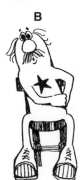

Exercise   HAMSTRING STRETCH (BACK OF THIGH)

1 Sit in a chair with a second chair facing you.
2 Put one leg up on chair.
3 While keeping back straight, slowly bend at the hips until stretch is felt in back of thigh.
4 Return to starting position.

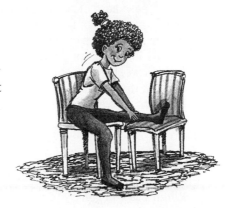

 Exercise   QUADRICEPS STRETCH (THIGH STRETCH)

1 Can be performed standing or lying down.
2 Grab ankle or pant leg and pull heel toward buttock until a stretch is felt in front of thigh.

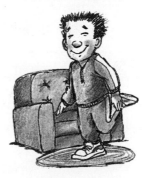

 Exercise   CALF STRETCH

1 Can be performed off step, curb, or tread-mill.
2 Start with both feet on step.
3 Drop one heel at a time off edge, keeping back leg straight.
4 To vary this exercise, perform with back leg slightly bent.

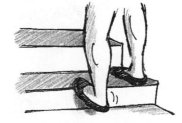

STRENGTH TRAINING

Strength training is another important component of your overall physical fitness program. Strength training may increase muscle strength and endurance, increase ease of activities of daily living, improve posture, decrease risk of injury, maintain or increase bone health, and improve how you look.

There are many ways to strength train. You can use free weights, weight-training machines, pulleys, or resistive bands/tubing. Perform strength training 3 days per week. A day of rest is needed for recovery before repeating the same workout. Include weight-training exercises for both sides of the joint. Lift the weight slowly and with control while maintaining the muscle tension. Do not hold your breath while strength training. Coordinate lifts with breathing.

This is a suggested way of progressing your strength-training program:

1. Initially perform 5 repetitions and increase up to 10 repetitions.

2. When you can complete 10 repetitions of the strengthening exercises, gradually increase to 15 to 20 repetitions.

3. When you can complete one set of 15 to 20 repetitions of the strengthening exercises, increase weight by 1 pound increments and return to step 1.

Upper Body Strength Training

 Exercise SHOULDER PRESS

1 Sit in a straight-back chair with your feet slightly apart.

2 Start with elbows bent and hands at shoulder level with palms facing forward.

3 Slowly extend arms above head until elbows are almost straight.

4 Return to starting position.

A   B

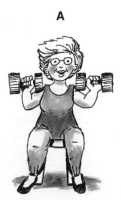 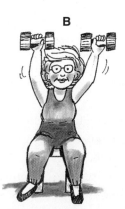

Exercise DIAGONAL ARM RAISES

1 Sit in a straight-back chair with your feet slightly apart and your arms crossed in your lap.

2 Lift your arms upward and out in a straight diagonal.

3 Return to the starting position.

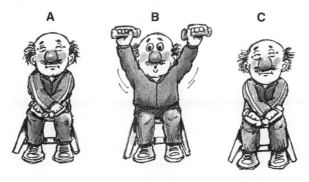

A   B   C

 Exercise SIDE ARM RAISES

1 Sit in a straight-back chair with feet slightly apart and arms down at your sides.

2 Lift your arms out and up until they are at shoulder level.

3 Return to the starting position.

(For variation, this exercise may be performed by lifting your arms out to the front of your body.)

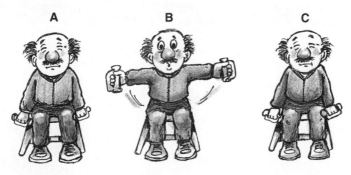

A   B   C

Exercise ARM CURL

1 Sit in a straight-back chair with feet slightly apart.

2 Start with arms hanging straight down by your sides and palms facing forward.

3 Bend elbow and "curl" weight up toward shoulder, while keeping elbows tucked in to sides.

4 Return to starting position.

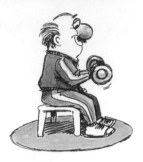

Lower Body Strength Training

 Exercise SITTING HIP FLEXION

1 Use ankle weights or place resistive bands around thighs.

2 Flex hip by lifting thigh straight off chair.

3 Return to starting position.

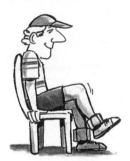

 Exercise SITTING LEG EXTENSION

1 Secure ankle weights or resistive bands around ankles.

2 Straighten and bend knee.

3 Return to starting position.

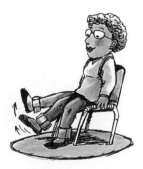

Exercise STANDING LEG CURLS

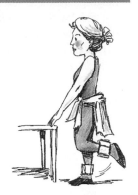

1 Secure ankle weights or resistive bands around ankles.
2 Stand up straight with hands on table or chair for balance.
3 Keep a slight bend in supporting leg and keep thighs parallel.
4 Bend knee and bring foot back toward buttocks.
5 Return to starting position.

Exercises to Strengthen Abdominal Muscles

 Exercise ABDOMINAL CRUNCH

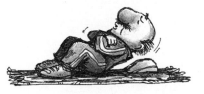

1 Lie on your back with knees bent and feet flat on the floor and cross your arms in front of your chest.
2 While exhaling, with eyes fixed on a spot on the ceiling, raise your head and shoulders.
3 Inhale and return to starting position.

 Exercise KNEE BENDING

1 Lie on your back with knees bent and feet flat on the floor.
2 While exhaling, bring the left knee toward your left shoulder and press the small of your back against the floor.
3 Inhale and return to the starting position.
4 Repeat on the right side.

A 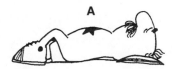 B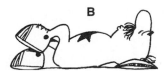

CONCLUSION

The importance of an exercise training program cannot be overemphasized. Exercise for people with lung disease has been shown to be beneficial. Exercise is an essential component of a healthy lifestyle. **Endurance, strength, and flexibility training** are the three components of your overall physical fitness program. Your doctor and other health care professionals can guide you. It is your job to get started on your exercise program and stay with it.

10

Letting Go: Relaxation Techniques

WHY TALK ABOUT RELAXATION?

When you are physically and emotionally relaxed, you avoid excessive oxygen consumption caused by tension of overworked muscles. Relaxation also decreases other undesirable manifestations of stress, such as mental irritability and anxiety that might induce bronchospasm, increased shortness of breath, and fatigue. By using some of the suggested relaxation methods outlined in the following sections, you can relieve the tension that increases your respiratory difficulties. Complete muscular relaxation is also important to gain maximal benefits from all other exercises.

The key to relaxation is, above all, breathing control. When you can master controlled breathing techniques, relaxation of the accessory muscles, and prolonged exhalation with pursed lips at times of stress, you have achieved a major victory in the battle against panic. At such times you should also remember positioning, which can be either standing or sitting, but always leaning forward with your arms supported.

To achieve the maximum benefit, relaxation techniques should be practiced on a regular basis. There are tapes of relaxation exercises that you can purchase at a local bookstore, or you can record your own tape with background music. Some people prefer to listen to calming music and follow the head-to-toe sequence described below.

To practice this first progressive relaxation technique, lie down on a comfortable surface and place one pillow under your head and one under your knees. Having quiet, peaceful surroundings is helpful. The principle that applies here is that maximal relaxation follows maximal contraction. Always tighten and relax the muscles gradually.

Head and Neck

1. Pull your chin down toward your chest as tightly as possible and push the back of your head into the pillow, then let go.
2. Turn your head from side to side in a relaxed manner.
3. Let it stop when it comes to a comfortable position

Shoulders

1. Shrug your shoulders and tighten the shoulder muscles as much as possible.
2. Let go.

Arms

1. Do one hand and one arm at a time.
2. Bend your elbow and make a fist out of your hand. Tighten as much as possible, then let go.
3. Straighten your arm and fingers. Tighten as much as possible, then let go.

Legs

1. Do one leg at a time.
2. Straighten your leg and point your toes; tighten as much as possible, then let go.
3. Pull your toes toward your nose and push your heel and the back of your leg into the bed.
4. Tighten as much as possible, then let go.

Back

1. Arch your back up in that slow, easy way that a cat does.
2. Do not lift your hips while arching. Tighten as much as possible, then let go.

Face

1. Tighten (scrinch) all of your face muscles.
2. Hold, then let go.

Eyes

1. Try to focus your eyes on something. Watch it and slowly let your eyelids grow heavy.
2. Open your eyes and let them close gradually until they feel comfortably closed. Sweet dreams!

OTHER RELAXATION TECHNIQUES

Another way to control your tension is to create in your mind a mental picture of something that gives you a good and comfortable feeling. This may be a scene, real or imagined: a landscape with rolling hills, green grass, and trees with their leaves gently moving in the wind; the beach; a poolside; or your mother's kitchen. Try to make your mental picture detailed. Each time you find yourself in a difficult situation that you cannot immediately leave (for example, a crowded elevator), use the visual image you have created as a mental escape. This will help keep your anxiety and shortness of breath under control until you can physically remove yourself from that situation.

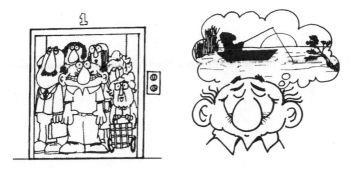

"Mind-over-matter" relaxation techniques are another way to help increase your mind's awareness and control over your body. There are many different ways to do this type of "self-hypnosis." You can simply concentrate on a certain part of your body; for instance, concentrate on your right hand and envision that it is becoming very limp, soft, heavy, or light. Any of these sensations will induce relaxation. Sometimes during a stressful or anxiety-provoking event, blood will rush to the central organs in the body, leaving the limbs cool and moist. Thinking of your hands and feet as "getting warm" is very effective, since relaxation will occur when the temperature increases. Try it first with one hand and, when you have succeeded in warming it, proceed up the arm, to the shoulder, then to the other hand, and so on until you have finally "told" your whole body to relax and it has obeyed you.

Another useful relaxation technique is one most frequently used in different types of meditation. Concentrate on one word and repeat it over and over to yourself (such as the word *free*). Repeat the word each time you breathe out. Do not let yourself get distracted by intruding thoughts; ignore them and return to repeating your word. Don't be concerned about how deep a relaxation level you are reaching. When trying these different modes of relaxation exercises, become passive and allow relaxation to come about at its own pace.

Sleep eradicates the effects of daily fatigue. Many people with chronic lung disease, however, have trouble sleeping, sometimes because of their medications. The events of modern life, in addition, frequently overload human faculties, causing exhaustion that may not be corrected by sleep. Meditation is thought to produce an extraordinarily deep rest and a stress release much more complete than sleep. It is particularly suit-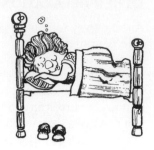ed for gradual removal of long-accumulated stress. This may be one relaxation method you will want to investigate further. Meditation can be used in conjunction with the progressive relaxation technique first mentioned. You start by relaxing your muscles, then you meditate.

Other modes of relaxation can include learning to give yourself a massage or having someone else give you one, especially on the neck and shoulder muscles. The vibrator you use for bronchial drainage can be very useful for this purpose also (see Chapter 8). Biofeedback is another way to learn to relax and explore your own ability to control tension and shortness of breath. You might have already found your own way to relax, be it soft music, yoga, or a bubble bath. There are many simple techniques worth trying. If they work for you, use them!

11

You Are What You Eat

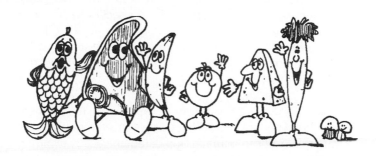

Eating is one of life's great pleasures. Food isn't just nourishment; it is associated with all types of significant events. What you eat may affect you emotionally and influence how well you function mentally. A healthful diet allows you to fight infection and disease and promotes a long and healthy life.

Nutrition and health are big business, and we are continually flooded with information. Newspapers, magazines, radio, and television have ads, articles, and commentaries about the subject. Some of the information comes from reliable sources; a lot of it does not. Nutrition is now "in." Whenever any health issue is popular, the public must be wary. People have to know *who* is saying *what*—and *why*. Daily there are stories that say "don't eat this" (it may kill you) or "do eat that" (it will cure whatever is wrong with you). One who reacts to all these stories can become confused at best and extremely anxious or sick at worst. Unfortunately, much of this information is incomplete or is based on either no scientific studies or a misinterpretation of the studies done. There is no question that good nutrition is important. There is also no question that there are well-meaning people who are convinced that eating sugar is "bad" or that taking large quantities of certain vitamins is "good." However, conviction, enthusiasm, and testimonials are no guarantee of scientific accuracy.

A sensible approach to nutrition begins with a basic understanding of how the body works and how it uses food to produce energy. The body and its digestive system are very smart. Most of the things you eat can be converted from one form to another by the body. It is very difficult to trick the digestive system. For example, the body requires sugar as an energy source. If you take none in, the body will make it out of other things you eat, or your "engine" will not run. Indeed, this ability of the digestive system to make the things it needs often saves us from ourselves when we go on strange fad diets. Given this marvelous, flexible manufacturing system, all we have to do to maintain good nutrition is to use common sense. Give the body an even break and it will serve you well. Therefore, the basic rule of good nutrition is a simple one: *eat everything in moderation*. Fad diets and fear of eating certain things are not warranted. Unless you have some kind of rare digestive disease, are truly allergic to some food (a very rare situation), have some kind of hereditary problem (again, quite rare), or have special medical problems, eating a regular, reasonably balanced diet is all you need to do. *Just avoid excesses*. Eating a gallon of ice cream a day does not make sense; nor does being terrified of eating a dish of ice cream. Salting foods until they are white is not moderation. There is no reason to challenge your body. Treat it reasonably. Eat things in moderation.

It certainly is a fact that with decreased physical activity, you need fewer calories to burn for energy; yet you still need protein, carbohydrates, fats, vitamins, and minerals. You can manage this balancing act by avoiding an excess of foods that provide mainly calories but few nutrients, such as sweets, fast foods, and packaged "goodies." Give some thought to your choices and select those foods that give you more of the nutrients you need.

An important goal for the individual with chronic lung disease is to maintain ideal body weight. This may not be the weight on the life insurance charts but the weight you felt best at and maintained through most of your adult life. Many of us gain extra weight in the midriff or stomach region. For the person with lung disease, this extra weight could mean increased shortness of breath because of the added pressure on the diaphragm. The diaphragm is the drumlike structure under the lungs that is responsible for much of the lungs' movement. Eating a large meal, consuming liquids during the meal, or eating foods that cause gas and distention may put pressure on the diaphragm, which causes difficult breathing. Being underweight can affect the ability to fight infection and cause fatigue. Discuss your dietary goals with your physician and dietician. They can provide information on weight maintenance for optimal health.

THE FOOD GUIDE PYRAMID: A GUIDE TO DAILY FOOD CHOICES

You can use the U.S. Agriculture Department's Food Guide Pyramid to follow a healthy diet by eating the recommended servings of grains, fruits, vegetables, meats, and dairy products each day.

The pyramid is divided into four horizontal layers containing the foods most common to the American diet. Just as a pyramid's strength comes from its wide base, the foundation of your total daily diet is built on a base of 6 to 11 servings of grains per day. The next layer is vegetables (3 to 5 servings) and fruits (2 to 4 servings). These two bottom layers are the foundation of the dietary pyramid. Meat and dairy products make up the third tier, with a recommendation of 2 to 3 servings each. Finally, the top section of the pyra-

THE FOOD PYRAMID

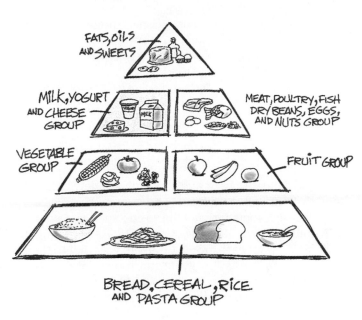

mid suggests limitation of added sugars and fats, which also are contained in some foods in each of the other food groups.

What counts as one pyramid serving? The following chart is a general guide. Combination foods, such as tacos, pizza, stews, and casseroles, often contribute servings from two or more food groups. To determine how much, the amounts of main ingredients must be estimated.

Food Group	Serving Size
Bread, cereal, rice, and pasta	1 slice of bread
	½ hamburger bun, bagel, or English muffin
	1 ounce ready-to-eat cereal
	½ cup cooked rice, pasta, or noodles
	½ cup cooked cereal
	2 to 4 crackers
	1 ounce pretzels
Vegetable	1 cup raw leafy vegetables (lettuce/spinach)
	½ cup cooked vegetables
	½ cup chopped raw vegetables
	¾ cup vegetable juice
Fruit	1 medium fruit (apple/banana/orange)
	½ cup berries or cut-up fruit
	½ cup cooked or canned fruit
	¾ cup fruit juice

Food Group	Serving Size
Milk, yogurt, and cheese	1 cup milk 1 cup yogurt 1½ ounces natural cheese 2 ounces process cheese
Meat, poultry, fish, dry beans, eggs, and nuts	2 to 3 ounces cooked lean meat, fish, or skinless poultry Count as 1 ounce meat equivalent: 1 egg or ¼ cup fat-free, cholesterol-free egg alternative ⅓ cup nuts ½ cup cooked dry beans 2 tablespoons peanut butter

By using the Food Guide Pyramid and choosing a variety of foods, including low-fat alternatives, such as lean meats and skim milk, you easily can follow a healthy daily eating program that will provide adequate amounts of calories, vitamins, and minerals. Record your food intake for 3 days and average the number of servings for each group. Compare your diet to the Food Guide Pyramid. Make changes to improve your nutritional intake. This is an easy way to ensure you are taking in a wide variety of nutrients to meet your needs without having to count calories and fat grams.

THE SIX BASIC NUTRIENTS

There are six nutrients that are necessary for health: water, carbohydrates, protein, fat, vitamins, and minerals.

Water

Water is responsible for approximately two thirds of your total weight. It not only helps to digest food and eliminate waste, but, for persons with lung disease, it also helps to keep mucus and secretions thin. Mucus that accumulates in the airways is a breeding ground for infection. If you are underweight, choose liquids high in calories, such as milk shakes and fruit nectars. If you are overweight, water is always a good choice. The person with chronic lung disease should drink 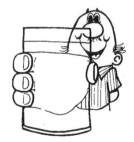 eight to ten glasses of fluid per day. When adding up your fluid intake, don't include beverages with alcohol or caffeine, because both cause you to lose fluid. You needn't worry about increased mucus from dairy products; there is no evidence that milk products produce mucus in lung tissue.

Carbohydrates

Carbohydrates are your body's preferred choice to make energy. They come in two categories: simple and complex. Simple carbohydrates are sugary type "treats"; complex carbohydrates include whole grains, breads, cereals, rice, and pasta. Complex carbohydrates contain many vitamins and minerals and the fiber essential to good health. Make them your frequent choice and consume simple carbohydrates only on an occasional basis.

Protein

This group provides essential amino acids the body uses to repair and maintain tissue. Dairy products, fish, poultry, and meat are good choices. Choose the low-fat varieties and trim any visible fat. Beans and legumes are also good sources of protein when combined with whole grains. This combination provides a complete protein source that is low in fat and high in fiber.

Fat

Fat contains "essential fatty acids," which must be supplied by the diet. It's easy to consume enough fat; however, some choices are better than others. The best choices are the monounsaturated fats that include canola, olive, and peanut oil. These fats are the least likely to raise blood cholesterol levels. Polyunsaturated fats are the next best choice. Saturated fats—the "hard fats" that include the marbling in beef, lard, tropical oils, butter, and margarine—are the least desirable. They have the greatest potential for increasing cholesterol levels.

Vitamins

Vitamins help to turn food into energy. Their functions vary widely and are essential to health. Here's a list of some of their functions:

- Vitamin A is important for growth and vision and to fight infection. Beta-carotene, a pigment found in the plant kingdom, is converted to vitamin A in the body. Good sources of vitamin A or beta-carotene include liver, dark leafy greens, and any yellow-orange vegetables.
- The B vitamins are important for nerve function, digestion, appetite, healthy skin, and conversion of carbohydrate to energy. Some good sources are whole-grain products, meat, poultry, fish, nuts, and dairy products.
- Vitamin C is important, but the amount needed is still in question. Some excellent sources include oranges, grapefruits, strawberries, broccoli, cantaloupe, and potatoes. Eating at least five servings of fruits and vegetables per day assures a healthful intake of this vitamin.

- Vitamin D is produced when the human body is exposed to sunlight. Most dairy products and dry cereals are fortified with vitamin D. Some other good sources include sardines, fresh salmon, canned tuna, and shrimp.
- Vitamin E is also a controversial supplement. Like vitamins A and D, it is a fat-soluble vitamin and is stored in tissue. It's always a good idea to check with a dietician or physician before adding supplements to your diet. Good sources of vitamin E include vegetable oils, nuts, wheat germ, and legumes.

Minerals

Minerals help maintain vital body functions and help manufacture bones, blood, and teeth. Some medications taken by people with chronic lung disease can interfere with absorption of calcium. Calcium is especially important for women, who are at greater risk of loss of bone mass as they age (osteoporosis). Dairy products provide the best sources of calcium. Check with your physician regarding your drug-nutrient interactions.

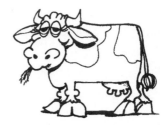

Vitamins and minerals are essential to good health and can easily be provided by a varied and balanced diet. Always be wary of supplement advertisements making unrealistic promises. Not only are supplements expensive—they can be dangerous.

Eating well is important to everyone, but the person with chronic lung disease has special needs. Some potential nutritional problems and solutions are included in the following section.

GAS AND DISTENTION

Eating too much at one sitting or eating certain gas-producing foods can cause a "bloated" feeling, put pressure on the diaphragm, and make breathing difficult.

SOLUTION:

1. Eat several small meals each day instead of three large ones. Drink fluids between meals rather than with meals. Eating small meals requires less energy expenditure.
2. Limit gas-forming foods. Some common offenders include:

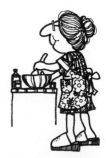

Apples	Carbonated drinks
Beans/legumes	Cauliflower
Beer	Onions
Broccoli	Radishes
Brussels sprouts	Sauerkraut
Cabbage	Sweets
Cantaloupe and other melons	Watermelon

3. Eat slowly and talk less during meals to avoid swallowing air. Don't exercise right before or right after eating. Consumption, digestion, and absorption of food require a significant amount of energy. Rest after eating.

LOSS OF MUSCLE MASS

Patients with lung disease often experience muscle wasting. A consistent exercise program helps preserve muscles and fight fatigue, and it can increase your energy level. Combine a healthful diet with exercise.

SOLUTION:

1. Eat a varied and balanced diet. Emphasize fruits and vegetables (at least five servings per day).
2. Eat at least two servings of protein-rich foods per day (for example, two 3-ounce servings of meat, fish, or poultry). Beans/legumes and dairy products are also good choices.
3. Increase the protein and calorie content of your food by adding nonfat dry milk to sauces, gravies, cream dishes, casseroles, and desserts. You can add approximately ¼ cup of nonfat dry milk to many recipes without changing the flavor. Increase the protein and calorie content of milk by adding nonfat dry milk to regular milk; just mix well and chill.

LOSS OF APPETITE

Many people with chronic lung disease experience loss of appetite and weight loss. If you are underweight, it is important to keep track of your weight and strive for weight maintenance. Mucus production and some medications can also decrease appetite.

SOLUTION:

1. Take medications with milk or meals unless otherwise advised.
2. Practice bronchial drainage an hour or two before meals.
3. Enjoy some fresh air and light exercise a short time before meals.
4. Prepare foods *you* enjoy that have enticing aromas. Vary your menus.

5. Celebrate your meals. Provide music, color, and outdoor locations for eating. Vary the colors and textures of your food.

6. Share your meals with a friend or loved one.

7. Take advantage of community meal programs at churches and senior centers.

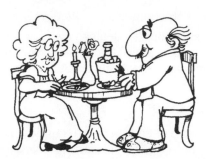

POTASSIUM DEPLETION

People with chronic lung disease may have low potassium levels. This may be due to diuretics (water pills), but usually the cause is unknown. Some signs of low potassium levels are weakness, tingling, numbness of the fingers, and leg cramps.

SOLUTION:

Consume foods high in potassium every day. Here are some examples:

Bananas	Mushrooms	Spinach
Broccoli	Oranges	Tomato products
Dried fruit	Peanuts	Winter squash
Dry skim milk	Potatoes	Yams

FLUID RETENTION

Foods high in salt (or sodium) often cause fluid retention. If you retain water or have high blood pressure, you may need to decrease the amount of salt in your diet. Salt is the most frequently used additive in the United States and is contained in almost all processed, canned, and fast foods. A dietician can provide helpful information on reducing sodium intake.

TIPS TO SAVE TIME AND ENERGY

Preparing meals can leave you fatigued, with little energy to enjoy your meal. Here are a few suggestions to make meal preparation easier:

1. Make one-dish meals (casseroles). These are easy to prepare and clean up.
2. Prepare large quantities and freeze in individual "packages" for future meals.
3. Pace yourself while cooking. Try not to rush when preparing a meal.
4. Use conveniences like a microwave or Crock-Pot. These appliances can help you make more nutritious meals than you could by the conventional methods. Oven cooking requires less energy than stove top cooking.

IN CLOSING . . .

Check with your physician or dietician before taking supplements or trying a new dietary regimen. The goal is to eat healthful, nutritious food 80% to 90% of the time and to be aware of the foods you consume. There is an abundance of food available; with minimal planning and effort, your meals can be a great source of pleasure while simultaneously providing strength, nourishment, and energy.

Good Luck!   Good Health!   Good Eating!

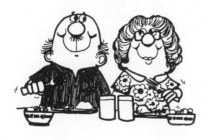

12

You Don't Have to Be Grounded: Leisure Fun, Recreation, and Travel

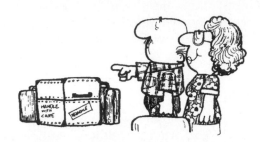

Activities away from the home are an important part of life for most people, whether for business or for pleasure. Stimulating, exciting, restful, and fun leisure time or recreation—these are the things dreams are made of. Most people dream of the day they can spend their time leisurely doing whatever they want, whenever they choose. People with lung diseases are no different. The time to get up and go . . . is now!

Where would you like to be today? What would you like to be doing? Are there recreational things to do in, around, or near your home that are on your wish list? Many people with lung conditions feel stressed about entertaining or are afraid to leave the familiar safety of their homes for travel or vacation. The most important considerations for leisure activities are planning, allowing time to pace your activities to a comfortable breathing rhythm, allowing sufficient rest between times of exertion or excitement, and who else is around to help.

You may need to travel for business purposes, to visit with family and friends, or just to enjoy "getting away" and seeing new places (or pleasant old ones). But when you have a breathing problem, the thought of leaving the security of home may prevent you from venturing out. Questions of safety, getting sick, and needing help may arise. For most people with chronic lung disease, however, there are relatively few reasons not to travel. With desire, a little foresight, determination, and a little extra planning, you don't have to miss out on the pleasures of life or be grounded just because you have difficulty breathing!

You can take a vacation, but there is no vacation from health considerations or from respiratory care. You cannot tell your lungs that you are going on a trip and will return tomorrow or in 2 weeks to care for them. Although your daily routine will be interrupted, you must adhere as closely as possible to your health care routine. This means you must take your medications regularly, allow sufficient rest time, and maintain your fluid intake. If your routine includes breathing exercises and physical training exercises, they must be continued too.

The most important move you can make in planning a happy and healthful vacation is to consult your doctor, who may review your plan of care and indicate whether any part of your medical management program can be modified while you are away. Your doctor may want to give you the name of a physician at your destination whom you can contact if any difficulties arise. **You may even want to request a copy of your medical records to carry with you and perhaps have a copy sent ahead to a designated physician.** Your doctor can help you make an emergency medical plan, to be used while you are in transit or at your destination. This might also be a good time to discuss an advance medical directive "durable power of attorney for health care," so that YOU are making the decisions that your designee would abide by, in case of an emergency. (For more information see Chapter 15, "When to Call Your Doctor and What to Do in an Emergency.")

When planning for fun or choosing a vacation site, consider how these few items might affect your overall health, and particularly your breathing.

LOOK AT THE BIG PICTURE:

- How is your overall health and energy level?
- How is your stamina?
- Do you tire more easily than usual?
- Do you have any signs of an impending flare-up of your lung condition?
- Who can help with planning, preparing, and doing?
- What will you need to take with you?
- What will you need to do, to keep you healthy during the activity or vacation time?
- If you don't have your act together, don't take the show on the road!
- Get organized and get going!

INFECTIONS:

- Assess yourself carefully before leaving home for any sign of an impending infection.
- Are there any viral flu epidemics at your destination? (Of course, you should check with your doctor about obtaining a yearly flu vaccine, regardless of known epidemics.)
- Does anyone you are going to visit with have a cold or another kind of contagious illness? If so, you may want to reschedule your plans or trip.

AIR POLLUTION:

- How smoggy is the area?
- How are the pollen and mold counts?
- Will you have an air-conditioned room?
- Reserve nonsmoking accommodations.
- Avoid smoking areas whenever possible.

ALLERGY:

- If allergies play a part in your illness, avoid areas that have high levels of air pollution, pollens, or mold counts.

ALTITUDE:

- Consider the altitude of the areas that you will travel through and at your destination. As we ascend, there is less atmospheric pressure; closed air spaces in our bodies, like inner ears, intestines, and emphysematous lungs, expand and can make breathing more difficult. The air becomes less dense, and there is less oxygen available in each breath. At elevations slightly above sea level, this change may be insignificant. But in cities at higher altitudes (that is, a few thousand feet to a mile [5,280 feet] high) or during air flight (the cabins are pressurized to an atmosphere equal to about 1 mile high), the effect on people with chronic lung disease may be important, resulting in increased shortness of breath and other symptoms. Supplemental oxygen needs might be increased at higher altitude.

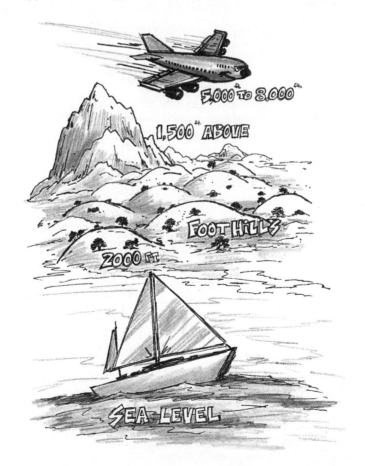

- Discuss with your doctor how different altitude changes may affect you. If you need supplemental oxygen at higher altitudes, you must take it with you or arrange to have it there when you arrive.
- If your doctor says that you will need supplemental oxygen while traveling, contact your travel carrier and oxygen equipment supply company in advance for assistance, requirements, and/or restrictions. Some carriers will require a written release from your doctor and a prescription for the amount of oxygen prescribed. If you currently use oxygen or other respiratory equipment, ask your local vendor for the name of a company that could assist you en route or at your destination. You may have to take some of your equipment with you, but arrangements can be made for whatever equipment or oxygen supplies you need to be waiting for you on your arrival. Don't forget your cleaning supplies! Your rehab team and local supplier can be of great help with these details.
- Most airlines will supply oxygen for you for the duration of the flight, but not during layover time on the ground. You might want to plan your trip so that any layover time is spent at sea level, to minimize oxygen needs while on the ground. The airline may require a written release from your doctor to travel and a specific prescription for the amount of oxygen to be used in flight. Some airlines won't allow oxygen use at all. Oxygen use charges are made by take-off and landing coupons, so nonstop might be less costly. It is possible to transport your own empty equipment on board, as luggage or freight, to be filled at your destination. Be sure to check the rules, and be prepared well in advance.
- Cruise ships, trains, and buses allow supplemental oxygen to be used, with a few caveats. Contact them early in the planning stage to learn their requirements.

CLIMATE:

- Changes in temperature, humidity, wind, pollution, and altitude can greatly affect your breathing comfort. Cold air can trigger bronchospasm (airway narrowing). Warm humid air, wind, pollution, and altitude may make it more difficult to breathe.
- Go prepared for climate and weather changes. Consider both indoor and outdoor climates. Some heating or air conditioning might seem extreme to your lungs.
- Take extra clothes to layer for warmth. Be prepared for possible changes in the projected weather conditions.

MEDICATIONS:

- Make a checklist of all of your medications. Include over-the-counter medicines, vitamins, and minerals.
- Take enough of each product, in its original container, to last you through the trip and for a few extra days in case of delay. Be very sure to take a suf-

ficient supply of your prescription medications if you are going to a foreign country.

- It is occasionally difficult to get prescriptions from one pharmacy or geographic area filled in another. Nevertheless, try to take typed and signed prescriptions from your physician as another possible safeguard.
- Discuss with your doctor having a "just in case" group of medications (e.g., antibiotics, steroids) that you might need to use if your condition worsens.
- When traveling to foreign countries, you may need a supply of general medicines with you (aspirin, antidiarrhea medicine, and others). The quality of medications is not the same throughout the world.
- Avoid unknown medications, especially over-the-counter preparations, since many of these contain substances that can cause harm.

EQUIPMENT:

- Check with your medical equipment supply company about taking your home care devices, equipment, and supplies with you.
- Ask your vendor to help you make arrangements with a company at your destination, if possible, or give you the name to contact before you leave home.
- Check to see if there are any additional adapters that will be required for your equipment. Special electrical connectors and converters may be needed for international travel.
- Take product information with you for repair and/or customs considerations.

YOUR ROUTINE:

- Establish a travel routine for your treatments, exercise, and equipment cleaning. Write it down and follow it carefully.
- Travel is tiring; allow time for frequent rest stops. Relax and enjoy yourself. Don't try to do too much in one day; get adequate rest and sleep.

HELPFUL RESOURCES:

- Talk to your doctors; they are your first resources.
- Call your local pulmonary rehabilitation program. They will be happy to share information and give assistance where they can.
- Your medical equipment supply company can offer lots of service.
- Consult your local American Lung Association and their *"Better Breathers Club" Travel Guide*.
- The American Association for Respiratory Care's *Breathin' Easy*, a travel guide for travelers with pulmonary disabilities, can be found on line at their web page www.aarc.org; then click on the "Breathin' Easy" logo or search for oxygen4travel.com.

**Fun leisure activities, recreation, and travel
make life interesting and rewarding.**

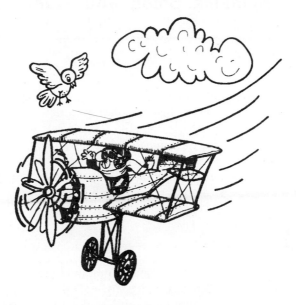

**Relax, Have Fun, Explore, and Travel whenever possible,
but plan ahead.**

13

Smoking, Smog, and Other Bad Stuff

Avoiding irritants is a good way to prevent further damage to your lungs. People with lung disease cannot live in isolation from the rest of the world, but they can make healthy choices and educated decisions.

The causes of lung disease are many and complex. Our understanding of the causes and what makes chronic lung disease worse is far from complete. We do know that inhaled irritants can adversely affect your lungs, and limiting exposure to these can help to maintain your lung function and prevent deterioration.

SMOKING

Today everyone knows that cigarette smoke impairs lung function. Cigarette smoke can paralyze the hairlike projections, called cilia, in the bronchial walls. As a result, the cilia cannot move mucus toward the throat, where it is eliminated. Smoke also irritates the cells in the bronchial walls that produce mucus. This irritation causes inflammation, an increase in mucus production, and chronic cough. Mucus that collects in the bronchial tubes impairs the movement of air and increases the likelihood of lung infections.

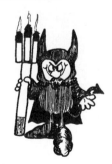

People with chronic lung disease, especially, should not smoke. If you are still smoking, seek help from your physician, local chapter of the American Lung Association, Heart Association, or Cancer Society. They may offer smoking cessation classes or other therapies that might assist you in your attempt to stop smoking. If you have tried to quit in the past, try again. Eventually you will succeed. It is important not to feel guilty or angry with yourself for smoking in the past. Negative feelings do not help you or your lung condition.

Lung cancer is another serious disease linked to smoking. Cancer-causing elements, known as *carcinogens*, are found in cigarette smoke. These chemical agents may cause normal cells to develop into cancerous ones. Statistically, smokers have a far greater chance of developing cancer of the lungs than do nonsmokers. Lung cancer has been a leading cause of death among American males for some years. The incidence of lung cancer among women has increased as the number of women who smoke increases.

People with lung disease who continue to smoke are engaging in behavior that limits any benefit obtainable from medical treatment. The benefits derived from smoking cessation are great. You may actually *improve* your lung condition! The risk of heart disease, cancer, and the development of further lung disease may be reduced. Coughing episodes and mucus production are likely to decrease. If nothing else, you will help to preserve the lung function you have. It's worth it!

ENVIRONMENTAL EXPOSURE

Environmental factors, such as temperature and humidity, may affect your breathing. There is no "ideal" climate or environment for all patients with chronic lung disease. The environment in which you feel most comfortable is the best one for you. Let's look at some environmental factors that may influence your breathing.

SECOND-HAND SMOKE

Second-hand smoke has been identified as a health hazard. Other people's smoke may actually harm your lungs and make you feel more short of breath. You should avoid smoke-filled places and let others know that smoke is harmful to you. Many smokers are not aware of the discomfort you may experience. Telling friends, "Yes, I do mind if you smoke" is especially difficult at first. With a little practice, it becomes easier. Here are some suggestions. Be polite and assertive when asking others not to smoke in your presence. A "No Smoking" sign on your door or desk may be sufficient. When exposed to smoke, seek out well-ventilated areas and avoid panic. Become proactive! Get involved with your local chapter of the American Lung Association and help educate people about the damaging effects of smoke.

AIR POLLUTION

Air pollution affects everyone, but research suggests that people with chronic lung disease may have more trouble breathing when air pollution levels are high. The four major pollutants are sulfates, ozone, particles, and carbon monoxide, primarily from factories and automobile exhaust. Carbon monoxide from car exhaust interferes with the blood's ability to carry oxygen. When polluted air is exposed to the hot sun, it becomes even more irritating.

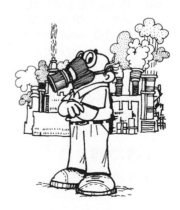

During "smog alerts," when air pollution rises to an unhealthful level, people with heart and lung disease are advised to stay indoors and avoid heavy exertion. Having air conditioning in your home may be helpful. Avoid rush hour traffic because of increased automobile exhaust. If you plan to travel, consider the air quality of the places you visit.

INDUSTRIAL POLLUTION

This occurs when the air in your workplace affects your breathing. It may be caused by dust, fumes, gases, and vapors from chemicals. Well-known industrial pollutants include asbestos and coal dust. We are discovering new forms of indoor pollution every day. Therefore, if you believe that the air in your workplace is contributing to or causing lung problems, you need to report it.

TEMPERATURE

Variations in temperature affect some people. Very cold air has been known to cause bronchospasm. Temperatures above 90°F can also affect your breathing and cause dehydration if you are not drinking enough fluids.

WET VERSUS DRY CLIMATES

The only person who can tell if a wet or dry climate is better for your breathing is you. You should visit both climates and compare your symptoms and how you feel.

ALLERGIES

True allergies are abnormal responses to materials that exist in the environment. For example, chopping onions makes everyone's eyes water; that is not an allergy but an irritation. It is sometimes difficult to distinguish between irritation and allergy. If you sneeze, develop a runny nose, have itchy eyes, or wheeze on exposure to certain things, you may have an allergy. It is best to avoid exposure to the allergen (substance that causes the reaction). When avoidance is not possible, allergies can be controlled with medicines such as antihistamines and corticosteroids. Discuss these possible allergies with your physician.

INFECTIONS

Infections of the lungs can be caused by viruses, fungi, or bacteria. People with lung disease often have more severe symptoms with infection because of decreased lung function. Therefore it is important to report symptoms of infection to your physician so that medical treatment can be started promptly.

Colds and influenza are caused by viruses. Annual immunization against influenza decreases the incidence of complications, hospitalization, and death due to influenza. Every year a new influenza vaccine is prepared. It provides protection against the influenza viruses expected to occur in the coming winter season. Patients with lung disease should receive a flu shot each fall, unless otherwise advised by their physician.

A "pneumonia" vaccine is also available to protect against certain types of bacteria that cause lung infection (pneumococci). Consult with your physician for the latest recommendations for receiving this vaccine.

Antibiotics are effective against bacteria and some fungi, and generally not against viruses. (New drugs that treat some viruses are now available.) Because bacterial infections may follow viral infections, patients with lung disease are often given antibiotics when they have cold or flu symptoms.

You should talk with your doctor about when and whether you should receive these vaccines or antibiotics.

14

The Psychology of Better Breathing

*If a man does not keep pace with his companions, perhaps it is because
he hears a different drummer.*

H.D. *Thoreau*

All of us would like to be able to do what we want, when we
want, and how we want. Unfortunately, we learn that many
factors impose limitations. How we deal with these limitations helps determine how happy, productive, and pleasant
our lives are.

Our state of health is one factor that can impose a significant limitation, and any chronic illness, such as chronic
lung disease, imposes limitations permanently. A chronic limitation can be
particularly difficult to deal with and can make individuals angry, anxious,
and depressed. Although this is understandable, it is unfortunate, because
the mind and body are closely interrelated. That is, physical health can influence mental health—and vice versa. This is particularly true for people with
chronic lung disease. Emotions can influence breathing in people with normal lungs, but they can have major effects on breathing when chronic lung
disease is present. Therefore dealing with your emotional or psychological
well-being is very important to your physical health.

Saying "Deal with your emotions" or "Learn how to live with limitations"
is easy; doing it is difficult. This chapter may help you by explaining the
emotional problems common to persons with chronic lung disease.

There are two kinds of problems you may face: how you view yourself and
how you relate to others.

YOU—THE PERSON WITH CHRONIC LUNG DISEASE

We all have a certain image of ourselves physically and emotionally. That image is critical to how we function and to how we relate to others, because our
self-esteem is based on it. Chronic lung disease may be associated with a
number of changes in physical image. You may gain weight because of inactivity or steroid medications, or you may lose weight because of decreased
appetite. You may have noisy breathing, or you may cough and produce sputum or phlegm. You may have to walk and do other things more slowly. You
may need to use oxygen in public. All of these things may impair your physical image and cause you to feel awkward, unattractive, or odd. If you feel

this way, you may think that others see you the same way, and your self-esteem may suffer.

In general, people have a lot to think about as they go about living every day. It is important to recognize that others are less likely to be focused on your physical appearance than you may think. If they do notice and ask questions, such curiosity on their part is normal. It can be satisfied by telling them the truth. You can calmly say, "It's all right, I have a lung condition and need to use oxygen" or "It makes me cough more than I would like." Most people understand and will easily accept the truth—and you. The people who count will accept you for what you are, not how you look. People who wear casts on their legs are always asked "What happened?" A straight answer usually ends the curiosity, and normal interpersonal relationships can resume.

Another limitation that can bother people with chronic lung disease is their vulnerability to things over which they have no direct control. All of us are vulnerable to a number of outside forces. But with chronic lung disease, many factors may pose a special threat to your well-being: infectious agents, atmospheric conditions, and environmental pollutants, for example. Such factors may lead to unpredictable changes in daily activities, which is irritating if you are used to being organized and to carefully planning your daily activities. When symptoms of shortness of breath and coughing vary, it can lead to a gradual loss of self-confidence. Some even find themselves avoiding commitments, such as going to dinner with friends or traveling, for fear they won't feel like going by the time the event rolls around.

Chronic lung disease may lead to other alterations that can impair self-esteem. You may need to modify your work schedule or seek early retirement. You may need to modify or eliminate certain pleasurable activities, such as tennis, golf, bowling, hiking, or other forms of recreation. You may need to move to seek a more favorable climate, causing you to leave behind friends and familiar surroundings. These changes can cause periods of depression, which practically all people with chronic lung disease experience.

Depression involves feelings of sadness, hopelessness, and worthlessness. The symptoms are subtle in the beginning, consisting of a lack of interest in things (possibly including your personal appearance, food, and outside activities) and fatigue. Often going out becomes a chore; friends and hobbies are abandoned. Everything becomes too much effort. Depression must be recognized early. Unless it is, the inactivity that results can worsen your condition. There is no easy antidote. You must force yourself to start moving, call friends, and go out; if necessary, seek professional help or counseling.

Certain phobias (abnormal fears of common experiences) may develop because of the real fear of becoming short of breath. For example, panic may be associated with entering closed spaces, even a shower stall. This panic worsens shortness of breath, and a terrifying vicious cycle of fear and further difficulty in breathing can result. This cycle can be prevented by learning how to control such situations with proper relaxation and breathing techniques. Pulmonary rehabilitation professionals can help you gain better control over these situations.

Another common response to chronic lung disease (or any chronic illness) is denial. It is certainly useful to avoid becoming totally preoccupied with yourself and your illness. But denying illness can be hazardous, especially if it leads to forgetting medicines, treatments, doctor appointments, and appropriate limitations on your activity. It may lead to hiding your limitations from other people. You need to strike a balance between living within your limitations and denying their existence.

HOW YOU RELATE TO YOUR SPOUSE AND SIGNIFICANT OTHERS

Pulmonary illness has an impact not only on you, but also on your significant others, because it often alters the roles you play in relationship to others. For example, in marriage each partner usually accepts certain responsibilities. Each partner comes to rely on the other for certain activities; one may deal with finances and with social arrangements; the other may deal more effectively with certain problems or people or with house maintenance or shopping. When pulmonary illness occurs, the nature of this sharing may need to change, either temporarily or permanently. Your spouse may have to assume new roles. There is danger in this situation for both the person with chronic lung disease and the spouse. Some people with lung disease may become more and more dependent on the healthier partner (who, in turn, may become essentially a full-time nurse). The one with chronic lung disease may fear being left alone and require more and more from the spouse, including giving up his or her outside activities and work. Both may resent the situation (often quietly)—one angry about being dependent, the other angry about becoming so depended upon. The answer is to discuss what is going on in the relationship. Excessive dependence (or doting) is to be discouraged. Both partners should do their share, even if those shares are modified in amount or nature.

Intimacy and Sexuality

To maintain an active, enjoyable sexual life, there are also certain changes that a couple may have to make when one member has lung disease. They may not be able to perform some of their previous sexual practices, since the extent of exercise tolerance may be diminished. The length of time spent in activities such as foreplay may have to be modified. In addition, certain positions previously used may no longer be comfortable and a change may

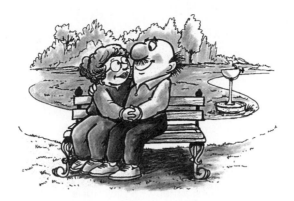

be necessary. But there is no way that modifications can be made in sexual activity unless the couple is open enough to talk about sex. Also, remember that there is more to an intimate and loving relationship than just the physical activities of sex.

An unfortunate type of communication that couples frequently engage in is a game called "I hope you can read my mind." That is, one partner wishes something would change in their sexual relationship and hopes that the spouse will comply with the unspoken wish. The ice may have to be broken by one person who just comes out and talks about it. As an example, one woman was required to use oxygen for any type of exertion, including sexual activity. She felt that having her oxygen tank in the bedroom detracted from the sexual atmosphere during relations with her husband. Her solution was to place the tank outside the bedroom and use a long tube that reached the bed. There is no reason for sexual activity to stop because a person has lung disease. The key is to be open about it, and then modify the activity to that which is physically possible.

Friends

If you have a negative image of yourself, it may interfere with your friendships. You may begin to fear that you are more trouble than you are worth— that you are a burden to others. Your response may be to withdraw from relationships or to try and maintain a facade (doing more than you should really do). Again, the fact is that your friends rarely share these same feelings (that you are a burden) and will respect and understand your limits. If you ask them to walk more slowly, to not smoke around you, or to alter social plans, almost all will understand and respond. But you can't play "read my mind." You must tell your friends about your limits rather than try to hide them. You can take an active role in planning your social life so that it fits within your limitations. There is no need to be totally left out.

THE BOTTOM LINE

We have reviewed some of the common problems faced by patients with lung disease and some of the feelings they may develop. There are some very important principles you must remember to help you maintain both a positive state of mental health and a good quality of life. First, having lung disease does not necessarily mean you must give up certain activities in your life. Instead, you should modify your activities and still be involved in them. Many people have difficulty learning to pace themselves, but with patience and practice, it can be done. For example, people who are distraught that they can no longer play 18 holes of golf may find that it is possible to play 9 holes with a cart. Patient and spouse can enjoy golf again—a pleasure they thought was gone forever. When you have lung disease, you may develop misconceptions as to the safe limits of physical exertion; that is, once you begin to develop shortness of breath, you may stop the activity instead of slowing it down. There is a tendency to stop sooner and sooner in the activity, and consequently to begin to feel that you can do very little. Although you may have to slow down, you can learn that if you push yourself a little, you can do more than you thought. Doing more will improve your self-esteem and endurance. The important thing is to figure out how you can do what you like. Don't give it up! Rearrange it! Adapt it to your needs! Soon the new pace will no longer be planned; it will become natural to you. You can continue to be involved with your family, with your friends, and with the world.

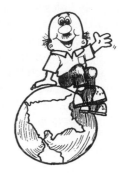

Another important principle is to learn as much as possible about your illness. You should try to learn about your lung function, your medicines, and your treatments. Ask questions of doctors, nurses, and therapists, as well as other people with chronic lung disease, until you have obtained answers. Participating in a pulmonary rehabilitation program can put you in touch with other people who know first hand your struggles and fears. Many people with lung disease find it comforting to meet others with similar needs. Spouses, significant others, and family members may also find it

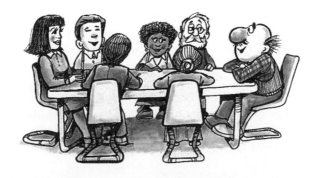

helpful. The process of educating yourself about your illness has enormous psychological value. As you know more about your illness, some of the unfounded fears can be dispelled. In addition, as you develop more understanding, you can play a more active role in keeping yourself healthy and helping yourself when you are ill. A great deal can be learned not only from medical personnel, but also from others with lung disease. People with chronic lung disease have accumulated a vast amount of experience about how to live successfully within the physical limits that exist. You can share their experiences, contribute your own, and give each other support. This can be done through rehabilitation programs, at American Lung Association meetings, and in informal groups.

The essence of good psychological health is to maintain a positive attitude toward living, while still knowing the facts and being realistic. Remain as active as possible, and try to maintain your sense of humor. Your life is not "over" because of lung disease; it is changed, but you can enjoy this changed life greatly if you maintain a positive image of yourself. Remember always to focus on what you *can* do, not just on what you *can't*.

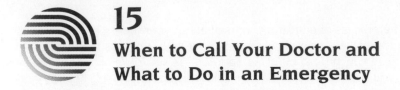

15

When to Call Your Doctor and What to Do in an Emergency

WHEN TO CALL YOUR DOCTOR

Most people with *chronic lung disease* have regularly scheduled visits with their doctor. But when should you call
your doctor between these visits? Usually, in discussions
with your doctor, details are worked out to cover this
question. In general, however, there are two major "signals" that your doctor will want to know about:

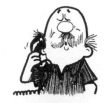

1. Any *change* in your symptoms, particularly if this
   change lasts more than 1 day
2. Any *new symptoms* that you develop

Obviously, we all have our ups and downs, our good days
and bad. But changes and new symptoms should be
called to your doctor's attention.

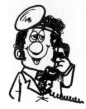

Some of the *changes* or *new symptoms* that might be important are:

- Fever
- Increased shortness of breath, added difficulty in breathing, or in-
  creased wheezing (more than usual)
- Increased coughing (more frequent, more severe, or both)
- Increased sputum production
- Change in color of sputum (to yellow, gray, or green)
- Change in consistency of sputum (thicker)
- Swelling of ankles, legs, or around eyes
- Sudden weight gain (3 to 5 pounds overnight)
- Palpitations of the heart or pulse faster than usual
- Unusual dizziness, sleepiness, headaches, visual disturbances, irri-
  tability, or trouble thinking
- Loss of appetite (more than usual)
- Dehydration (evidenced by concentrated urine and dryness of skin)
- Chest pains
- Blood in sputum, urine, or bowel movement

You should discuss these "signals" with your doctor, who may want you to
change your medicines or add new ones (for example, increase fluid intake
and/or start a preselected antibiotic for fever and increased cough). The
more thoroughly you work out these signals ahead of time, the better you

will be able to deal with these changes, and the less frequently you will have to call your doctor on an emergency basis. But when in doubt, check it out with your doctor.

WHAT TO DO IN AN EMERGENCY

Many patients and their spouses and/or family members want to know what to do in an emergency. There are three things that will make it rather simple to deal with this question:

1. Become familiar with what an "emergency" is.
2. Know what options for medical care are open to you.
3. Have a *plan*.

In general, an "emergency" is some *sudden change* or *new development* in your condition, particularly changes or new things that impair your ability to function or that frighten you. Sudden and/or severe chest pains or shortness of breath are the most common "emergencies" in patients with chronic lung diseases. Coughing up blood is another. So *sudden changes* in your condition and *new symptoms* of a major kind usually constitute a true emergency.

Of course, many patients with lung disease have mild changes that are frightening and may cause panic. Other sections of this book offer methods for dealing with panic. For example, if breathing becomes more difficult, you should assume a sitting position and lean forward slightly; pursed lip breathing usually helps, as may using relaxation techniques (see Chapter 10). Inhalation of a bronchodilator aerosol (see Chapter 5) is useful if the shortness of breath is caused by bronchospasm. You must learn how to deal with such episodes; discussions with your doctor about these and other maneuvers will help.

But what if the symptoms are severe, don't go away, or are new? This constitutes a true emergency. In this situation, most patients want to see their doctor *immediately*, and that is a good idea because he or she knows you best. But that may not be possible or even in your best interest in an emergency. The key to making an emergency plan is, again, a discussion with your doctor. You should determine when he or she is available (no one is available 24 hours a day, 7 days a week!); how you can contact him or her; and, if your doctor is not available when you try to contact him or her, what you should do. Many doctors have associates who "take calls" when they themselves are not available; some do not. If you cannot contact your own physician (or associates), what should you do—call an ambulance or the paramedics? If you do that, to what emergency facility should you be taken?

The answer to these questions will be different in different communities. In general, an "emergency" means you need prompt access to medical care. Obviously, it is an advantage if your doctor (or associate) is available to provide your medical history, even if he or she cannot be physically present.

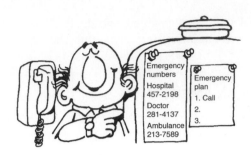

Therefore, the important thing is to *plan ahead* so you know what to do. Have a written "plan" near the telephone: *names of whom to call* and the *proper telephone numbers*: your primary doctor, "backup" doctors, ambulance or paramedic numbers, and location of the nearest emergency facility. Think through the situation ahead of time; put yourself in the place of your spouse or friend, as if you were helping *him or her* in an emergency. Once you have a plan, there is no reason for anyone to panic in an emergency. So worry about it *now* and get it worked out *now*. Hopefully, you will never need to put it into action!

Many patients don't want to "bother" their doctor; but whether your symptoms warrant "bothering" your doctor should be decided by the doctor. As you get to know each other and you become more knowledgeable, this decision will become easier. Err on the side of "bothering" whenever you are uncertain.

ADVANCE MEDICAL DIRECTIVES

Preparing in advance for a medical emergency allows you to maintain control of your health care decisions, regardless of what happens to you. The best way to do this is to put your preferences in writing, in the form of an advance medical directive. An advance medical directive allows you to set guidelines for health care decisions and to appoint a trusted family member or friend to act as your agent if you are no longer able to make decisions because of accident or illness.

The two most common advance directives are a living will and a durable power of attorney for health care.

Living Will

A living will is a written document that generally states the kind of medical care you want in case you are unable to make your own decisions. It is called a living will because it takes effect while you are still living.

Durable Power of Attorney for Health Care

A durable power of attorney for health care is a signed, dated, and witnessed paper that authorizes someone else to make your medical decisions if you are unable to make them yourself.

It is important to check the law in your state because some laws make it better to have one, the other, or both. Note that a living will does not allow you to name someone to make your medical decisions.

The first step is to decide what level of medical care you want and then protect your decisions by putting them in writing. Examine your values and attitudes toward health and disability. Consider how important independence and self-sufficiency are to you. How do you feel about your current health? Next talk to your doctor or health care provider about common treatments and their likely outcome. Some common treatments used for patients with lung problems are mechanical ventilation (breathing machine), use of medications to attempt to reverse a problem, or a feeding tube to provide nourishment. These treatments fall into three categories: life supporting, life sustaining, and life enhancing.

- Life support measures include cardiopulmonary resuscitation, use of respirator or ventilator, and medications.
- Life sustaining care involves treatment to prolong your life when your condition cannot be reversed or cured. Tube feeding and kidney dialysis are two treatments that fit into this category.
- Life enhancing care keeps you comfortable until death occurs naturally. Hospice care is comfort care that includes oxygen and pain medications.

Next understand what treatments can and cannot do, depending on your medical condition. Once you understand how specific therapies may affect your quality of life, you can decide which ones you want and which ones you would refuse. Some questions to consider are: Would you want treatment if it kept you alive but did not help you recover? What if the treatment could extend an acceptable quality of life for only a month? Should treatment keep you alive as long as possible?

Patients often say they do not want to be put on a machine to breath for them. It is important to understand that a mechanical ventilator does not treat your lung disease but is used to support your breathing during a crisis. Depending on the course of your illness, you may have a problem coming off the machine. In that case you have the legal right to limit artificial life support measures. If aggressive, curative treatment cannot improve the course of your terminal illness, comfort care is appropriate. Your doctor will help to relieve suffering in the final stages.

WHAT SHOULD YOU DO NOW?

- Talk to spouse, family, close friends, doctor, and clergy.
- Establish an advance directive, including your wishes regarding medical treatment. Your physician or health care provider will have the appropriate forms for your area.
- Discuss openly with your physician and family what to do if a crisis arises as you approach the final stages of your lung disease. Let them know your decisions.

If you do not want aggressive resuscitation, complete and post a "Do not resuscitate" form in your home. You can get this form from your doctor or Emergency Medical Services Agency within your county. After you complete the form, give a copy to your family members, agent, and doctor. Keep it close by. To be effective, an advance directive must be available for emergencies when you cannot speak for yourself. When medical professionals seek identification of an injured patient, it is normally found in a wallet or purse. Obtain a wallet card stating you have completed an advance directive, naming your agent, and indicating where your advance directive is located.

Decide whether you want to die in a hospital or at home. Investigate hospice care. Hospice care focuses not only on your medical needs but also on your emotional and spiritual well-being as well.

16

Getting It All Together

Developing a daily schedule can help you plan a workable, balanced regimen of treatments, rest, exercise, and recreation. Start by listing what you need to do each day. Include all the key elements of your particular program: medications, bronchial drainage, breathing exercises, aerosol treatments, arm exercises, walks, and snacks or small frequent meals.

It is important to set a realistic schedule to ensure a positive, successful outcome. You might have to push yourself at times as you work toward improving your strength and endurance, but the rewards will be worth the effort.

The sequence of your program is important. Here are some tips:

- Whatever time of day you have the most energy or feel the best is when you should exercise.
- Do not exercise or walk immediately after a meal. Wait at least an hour; or do your exercises before eating.
- Bronchodilators (medications that open your airways) should be used before bronchial drainage and, generally, before exercise.
- Bronchial drainage needs to be done before or at least 2 hours after meals.
- Remember to schedule rest periods, snacks, and fluids throughout the day.

An example of a typical daily schedule follows. With the help of your doctor, nurse, or therapist, fill in the blank schedule, using the example as a guide.

SAMPLE SCHEDULE
Morning

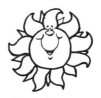

1. Take inhaled or nebulized bronchodilators.
2. If needed, perform bronchial drainage within 30 minutes of taking inhaled bronchodilator.
3. Have breakfast.
4. After at least an hour, walk at designated speed and for prescribed time. (Practice breathing exercises while walking.)
5. Have a nutritious snack with a glass of water.
6. Rest.

7. Have more liquids (space fluid intake throughout day and record the amount).

8. After you feel rested, do arm exercises, strengthening, and/or stretching exercises.

Afternoon

1. Have lunch.

2. Take medications, if prescribed.

3. After at least an hour, practice breathing exercises and relaxation techniques in a quiet setting.

4. Have a snack with a glass of water.

Evening

1. Have dinner.

2. Take medications, if prescribed.

3. An hour or so before bedtime, take inhaled or nebulized bronchodilator medication.

4. If needed, perform bronchial drainage within 30 minutes.

5. Clean nebulizer equipment (if applicable).

6. Perform relaxation techniques.

MODIFYING YOUR SCHEDULE

If you work outside the home, you can adapt your daily program of care. For example:

- You may need to get up earlier to allow plenty of time to do bronchial drainage. You may feel better if your lungs are clear of mucus.
- If bronchial drainage is not part of your program, you might choose to take your walk before getting ready for work.
- Arrange to take a short walk at lunch time, before eating.
- A good way to remind yourself to drink fluids throughout the day is to have a pitcher or thermos of water, juice, or other beverage readily available on your desk or nearby.
- At break time, find a quiet place where you can relax. Practice relaxation techniques or breathing exercises at this time.
- Practice breathing exercises periodically throughout the day while working.

Do not forget time for *activities you enjoy*. Arrange your schedule so that it includes time for your favorite hobbies and activities. These are important for your mental health!

YOUR DAILY SCHEDULE

Morning

1. _____
2. _____
3. _____
4. _____
5. _____
6. _____

Afternoon

1. _____
2. _____
3. _____
4. _____
5. _____
6. _____

Evening

1. _____
2. _____
3. _____
4. _____
5. _____
6. _____

17

You Don't Have to Do It Alone: Pulmonary Rehabilitation

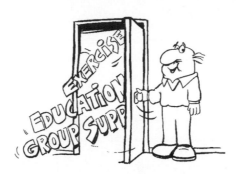

So far in this book we have discussed some general and specific health care measures that are important for persons with chronic lung disease. Learning more about lung disease and your own condition is an important step in improving your quality of life and helping you to cope better with it. Pulmonary rehabilitation programs can help you do this.

Rehabilitation is defined as "the restoration of the individual to the fullest medical, mental, emotional, social, and vocational potential of which he/she is capable." A *pulmonary* rehabilitation program is one that specializes in the rehabilitation of individuals with chronic lung disease. Pulmonary rehabilitation is a preventive health care program provided by a team of health care professionals. The primary goals of a pulmonary rehabilitation program are to provide you with the proper information, education, specific self-care therapies, and support to help stabilize your illness and improve your quality of life. People with chronic lung disease, like all persons, can live fuller and more productive lives if they participate *actively* in their own health care and have the *tools* with which to do so. Specific aims of pulmonary rehabilitation are as follows:

1. Teach patients, family members, and significant others about chronic lung disease, its effects and consequences, and ways to minimize or control the problems that chronic lung disease may cause.
2. Maximize physical strength and exercise tolerance.
3. Reduce symptoms and help you gain control over them.
4. Enhance emotional well-being.
5. Help you cope with the limitations and frustrations caused by having chronic lung disease.

6. Increase self-confidence and independence.

7. Help you develop a partnership with your physician and participate *actively* in your own health care.

WHAT ARE THE COMPONENTS OF A PULMONARY REHABILITATION PROGRAM?

Evaluation

Like any other person with chronic lung disease, you can participate in a pulmonary rehabilitation program if you are *motivated* to learn about your condition and to help yourself. An interview with a team member is the first step in the assessment process. During the interview, the program is explained, questions are answered, and medical records are reviewed. A specific program can then be designed to meet your individual needs.

Physical Therapy

Good bronchial hygiene, effective coughing, and bronchial drainage are taught as part of a self-care program. Instruction in proper breathing techniques and pursed lip breathing is provided. These measures are designed to reduce the work of breathing and to increase your ability to perform daily activities.

Respiratory Therapy Equipment

Instruction will be provided in the proper use and cleaning of respiratory therapy equipment, such as a metered dose inhaler, spacer, or nebulizer. The need for supplemental oxygen can be evaluated. If any equipment is needed, instruction will be provided regarding its proper use.

Education

An important goal of pulmonary rehabilitation is to help you and your family *understand* your disease and the kind of activities you can perform safely. Team members will discuss your medications and their side effects, proper nutrition, and how to identify signs and symptoms of a respiratory tract infection, among other topics. They will also teach you energy-conserving strategies, relaxation techniques, and how to reduce and manage stress.

Exercise

Exercise training has been shown to improve exercise capacity in persons with chronic lung disease and is an important component of pulmonary rehabilitation. After an initial evaluation, the team will determine a safe exercise program tailored to your needs. They will provide supervised exercise sessions and instructions for a home exercise program.

Feelings and Emotions

Successful rehabilitation requires attention not only to *physical* problems but also to *psychological*, *emotional*, and *social* ones. Understandably, persons with chronic illness often have difficulty dealing with the limitations and symptoms caused by their illness. One symptom in particular, *shortness of breath*, is closely linked to emotions. The sensation of shortness of breath may lead to anxiety and fear, which may then cause more shortness of breath and discomfort. This may cause a vicious cycle of inactivity and breathlessness. Support groups may help you to feel less isolated and alone. These groups also provide a forum in which you can share feelings, frustrations, hopes, and joys.

Benefits of Pulmonary Rehabilitation

Through the years, research has shown that there are definite measurable benefits from participating in a comprehensive pulmonary rehabilitation program. Some of these benefits include:

1. Increased knowledge about lung disease.
2. Increased exercise capacity.
3. Improved ability to perform activities of daily living.
4. Decreased sensation of shortness of breath.
5. Decreased anxiety and panic.
6. Improved quality of life.
7. Decreased time spent in hospitals.
8. Decreased use of health care services.

These benefits are certainly encouraging, but it must be stressed that it takes a motivated, committed person to participate in pulmonary rehabilitation and make the necessary lifestyle changes to improve his or her life. With a little help from a team of qualified, supportive, and caring health professionals, these benefits may be within your reach.

BEYOND COPD: RECENT ADVANCES IN PULMONARY REHABILITATION

Traditionally, the practice of pulmonary rehabilitation has focused on persons with COPD. Although patients with COPD represent a major subset of patients with chronic lung disease, there are patients with many other types of chronic lung disease who can benefit from pulmonary rehabilitation. The principles of rehabilitation can be successfully applied to many of these patients, including patients with restrictive lung diseases and cystic fibrosis as well as those undergoing treatments such as lung transplantation, lung volume reduction surgery, and cancer therapy. As in patients with COPD, rehabilitation goals should be tailored to meet the participant's individual needs. Education, exercise, and group or individual therapy provided by well-trained personnel will provide support and motivation for chronically ill and disabled persons. Pulmonary rehabilitation empowers patients to meet the daily challenge of living with a chronic illness.

Restrictive Lung Disease

Patients with restrictive lung diseases, previously described in Chapter 1, also experience shortness of breath at rest and with exertion that causes them to become sedentary and deconditioned. Participation in a comprehensive pulmonary rehabilitation program may help these persons better manage symptoms such as breathlessness, improve their knowledge of disease (including medications and oxygen or other treatments), and increase exercise tolerance. Patients with restrictive lung diseases often develop symptoms at a younger age and have to adjust to lifestyle changes earlier than many other persons with other chronic lung conditions. Anxiety and depression are common. Group or individual counseling is important and can be very helpful.

CYSTIC FIBROSIS

Cystic fibrosis (CF) is a genetic disease that commonly affects the lungs, pancreas, and sweat glands. In recent years, with improvements in medical care, the prognosis for persons with CF has improved dramatically. Shortness of breath and pulmonary complications are caused by mucus retention and recurring respiratory tract infections. As in other patients with chronic lung disease, exercise tolerance and the ability to perform activities of daily living can be improved by maintaining a regular exercise program. Exercise training can also help with clearing secretions and may be an appropriate addition to other forms of chest physical therapy. Although coughing spells may accompany vigorous exercise, coughing alone is not necessarily a reason to discontinue exercise. Each patient should be assessed individually to develop a safe and effective program. In addition, persons with CF lose more salt during exercise and should pay careful attention to fluid replacement, especially when exercising in the heat. Weight loss may be also a concern because of the effects that the disease can have on the digestive system as well as the lungs. Adequate nutrition is important, especially with any increase in caloric expenditure through exercise. Strength training is also an important component in the overall physical fitness program and can contribute to weight gain and increased strength.

Before and After Lung Surgery: Transplantation and Lung Volume Reduction Surgery

LUNG TRANSPLANTATION

Lung transplantation has become an increasingly available option for selected persons with severe disability from chronic lung diseases such as COPD, restrictive lung diseases, cystic fibrosis, and diseases of the pulmonary blood vessels (pulmonary hypertension). Pulmonary rehabilitation can be very helpful in both the preoperative period to prepare patients for surgery and in the postoperative recovery period after surgery.

In the preoperative period, which may last for a year or more while awaiting a lung transplant, pulmonary rehabilitation goals include preparing patients for surgery and optimizing their physical function and emotional well-being. Patients begin an individualized exercise training program designed to build strength and endurance, increase physical activity levels, and improve emotional well-being. The progression of the disease is monitored during the waiting period, and any changes are reported promptly to the transplant team. Patients have varying levels of knowledge about their illness and self-care techniques. The rehabilitation program can be used to teach techniques of chest physiotherapy, bronchial drainage, and breathing retraining and also to answer questions about the upcoming surgery and begin discussions about future concerns. Staff can assist patients in identifying signs and symptoms of a respiratory tract infection that needs to be diagnosed and treated early. Psychological support is ongoing and helps patients and family members cope with emotional and social stresses. Many patients report that this waiting period feels like their "life is on hold." The ability to interact with others awaiting transplantation provides significant benefit and group support to patients and families who are coping with the uncertainty of living with a serious illness and an uncertain future while awaiting the lung transplant.

After lung transplant surgery, the goals of pulmonary rehabilitation are similar but with a different focus. Patients will find that they can significantly improve their exercise capacity with reconditioning of their muscles, heart, and cardiovascular system. A gradual increase in exercise workload is prescribed. Continued education reinforces skills of self-assessment, such as home monitoring of blood pressure, pulse and other vital signs, lung function, and symptoms, and provides guidance about appropriate management. Emotional and social support is important as patients adapt to a "new condition," that of having a lung transplant instead of their chronic lung disease. New and different physical and psychological stressors develop after transplant. Patients may no longer be considered disabled and may risk losing disability income and benefits. Patients may also feel pressure to return to work but may not be able to perform their previous job, and potential employers may be reluctant to hire them because of uncertainty about their future health.

LUNG VOLUME REDUCTION SURGERY

There has been renewed interest in the surgical removal of diseased lung tissue in patients with emphysema through a procedure called lung volume reduction surgery (LVRS). Currently, this should still be considered an experimental therapy, and the role of LVRS for persons with emphysema is still under study. It has been suggested that pulmonary rehabilitation may be very beneficial for persons considering this operation. After rehabilitation, patients have a better understanding of their disease and its management and are in a better position to make an informed decision. For those who may choose to undergo LVRS, pulmonary rehabilitation helps to prepare patients for surgery and facilitate their recovery after the operation.

LUNG CANCER

Persons with lung cancer have both physical and psychological symptoms, not only from the cancer itself but also from any underlying lung disease, such as COPD. Also, such treatment options as surgery, radiation, or chemotherapy may increase symptoms of fatigue, weakness, or breathlessness. Therefore patients with already limited lung function may reach a lower functional status as a result of treatment. To facilitate recovery after surgery or other treatment(s), an individually tailored pulmonary rehabilitation program may help to provide strategies for symptom management, supervised exercise training, breathing retraining, nutrition counseling, respiratory therapy techniques, and emotional and social support, among others. Such programs are best administered when a patient is stable.

WHERE ARE PULMONARY REHABILITATION PROGRAMS LOCATED?

Pulmonary rehabilitation programs exist now in many parts of the world. Ask your physician, friends, other people with chronic lung disease, the American Lung Association, or the American Association of Cardiovascular and Pulmonary Rehabilitation for information on programs in your area. You may also refer to the resource chapter (Chapter 18) in this book on how and where to get started.

When you are ready, there are programs ready for you!

18

Resources: Where to Go for Information

You have read about chronic lung disease, what you can do to help yourself, and tips about how to manage your disease. What if you need more information? Where can you go?

The learning does not have to stop here. This chapter will provide you with information about public resources you can access to further your education and tips about how to find support within your community.

COMMUNITY RESOURCES

Your local American Lung Association (ALA) chapter is a great place to start. The ALA can provide you with credible and reliable information about many lung diseases and problems. It can also help you get involved with patient support groups, like the Better Breathers Club. The American Cancer Society is another national organization with local chapters that provide education and patient support groups.

You may be able to find senior centers in your community or support groups affiliated with local hospitals or other health care organizations that can provide you with social activities for people with conditions like yours and high-quality continuing education. Your local junior college or YMCA may have education and exercise classes tailored to your needs that you can enroll in. There are many community resources. One should be right for you.

THE INTERNET

The Internet is the largest resource of information. The Internet is a network that connects computers around the world. This network can support services for communicating, browsing, searching, and publishing. Information on the Internet is easily accessible by connecting to websites that are places you can visit with your computer. If you do not have a computer, you can purchase one that comes with all the necessary hardware and software to connect to the Internet. A computer vendor can provide you with instruction about how to use the computer. You can also go to your local library, many of which have computers available for public use.

On the Internet, you can find information on just about any topic you can imagine, including lung diseases. You can access this information from the comfort of your own home. There are many websites with health information, and it is sometimes difficult to tell just how accurate or reliable the information is. Knowing the purpose of a website can help you decide how credible it is. Websites may be there for different purposes, including selling products; providing support and discussion forums; or providing news and information.

Some websites are commercial and sell products. Like other businesses or advertisers, some of these websites may make health claims that may not be supported by scientific research or backed up by medical evidence. Some websites can also be a convenient way to purchase products without leaving your home. For instance, www.drugstore.com sells drugstore products and fills prescriptions online.

Websites that provide support to patients and their families via news and discussion groups or online chat rooms are a great way of getting in touch with others who have diseases or conditions similar to yours. Participants in these websites can offer support, understanding, and empathy with what you are going through. These support groups are places where participants can express their opinions openly. The purpose of most of these support groups is not to provide accurate medical information but to provide a place for people to express their feelings or concerns, seek advice, and support others. Because you may not know the people or how accurate the medical information is on these websites, it is important to discuss any medical advice or information from these Internet support groups with your own physician or health care provider.

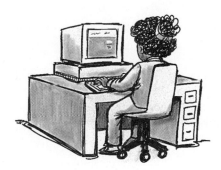

The following websites have online support and discussion groups for people with lung diseases and their families:

- Cardiothoracic Surgery Network—
  www.ctsnet.org/discuss/
- Chronic Lung Disease Forum—
  www.cheshire-med.com/programs/ pulrehab/forum/cldforum.html
- Emphysema Foundation for Our Right to Survive (Efforts)—
  www.emphysema.net

Many websites provide current news and information about health, diseases, treatments, and resources. These websites may have up-to-date information about the latest in medical research. They can also provide you with very comprehensive information about specific diseases and medical conditions, including symptoms, prevention, causes, diagnoses, and treatments. Be careful! Do not try to diagnose or treat yourself. If you learn about a medical condition, share your concerns and information with your health care provider. The following is a selected list of websites that provide health and medical information:

Health and Medical Information

- Dr. C. Everett Koop, former U.S. Surgeon General—
    www.drkoop.com
- WebMD—
    www.webmd.com
- Daily Lung—
    www.dailylung.com

Societies and Organizations

- American Lung Association National website—
    www.lungusa.org
- American Cancer Society—
    www.cancer.org
- American Association for Cardiovascular and Pulmonary Rehabilitation (AACVPR)—
    www.aacvpr.org
- The Alliance for Lung Cancer Advocacy, Support, and Education, (ALCASE)—
    www.alcase.org
- American Association for Respiratory Care (AARC)—
    www.aarc.org
- American Association for Retired Persons—
    www.aarp.org
- American College of Allergy, Asthma, and Immunology (ACAAI)—
    www.allergy.mcg.edu
- Medical Education Resources (MER)—
    www.mer.org
- National Emphysema Foundation (NEF)—
    www.emphysemafoundation.org
- National Lung Health Education Program—
    www.nlhep.org
- The Pulmonary Education and Research Foundation (PERF)—
    www.perf2ndwind.org

Government Websites

- National Institutes of Health (NIH)—
    www.nih.gov
    - National Heart, Lung, and Blood Institute (NHLBI)—
        www.nhlbi.nih.gov
    - National Cancer Institute (NCI)—
        www.nci.nih.gov
- The Agency for Healthcare Research and Quality (AHRQ)—
    www.ahrq.gov
- Medicare—
    www.medicare.gov

Accessing the resources in your community and on the Internet is a great way to continue the learning process. You will be able to stay current in your knowledge and learn about new developments in medical research, health care, and products to assist you in your daily life.

REMEMBER: INFORMATION IS POWER.

Get it! Use it!

19

A Look to the Future

Medical research is constantly working toward the answers to many of the mysteries
about lung diseases. Research is the key
to unraveling the mysteries of how the
lungs—and the rest of the human body—
work. Once we understand how the body
works, we are better able to figure out what
goes wrong in disease.

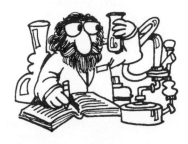

In cases of COPD, research on emphysema has indicated that the destruction of elastic tissue in the air sacs probably results from digestion of
this tissue by an enzyme called *elastase*. This enzyme is normally carried
around the body in white blood cells. We also know that a blood protein
called alpha-1-antitrypsin (also called alpha-1-proteinase inhibitor or alpha-
1-Pi or just a-1-Pi) can *inhibit* (prevent, block) the effects of elastase. Some
persons have an inherited deficiency of alpha-1-Pi and get emphysema early
in life, but this deficiency is rare. A-1-Pi has been purified and is now available to give to persons born with this deficiency. Why the elastase-inhibitor
system becomes unbalanced in patients who do not have a *hereditary* a-1-Pi
deficiency is not clear. It is known that oxidants, including those in cigarette
smoke, can render a-1-Pi *inactive*. Intensive research is focused on whether
this inactivation, and other factors, lead to lung injury. If we learn this, we
should be able to develop drugs to prevent this injury. Indeed, new drugs
that block elastase and oxidants are under development.

The causes of chronic bronchitis also are being studied. Clearly, there is
an association between cigarette smoking and certain industrial exposures
and lung injury—but why? What inhalants are responsible? What makes the
bronchial tubes behave the way they do? Can we develop drugs that will thin
mucus effectively or prevent excess mucus production or stop the inflammation of the bronchial tube lining? We probably can and will.

Existing drugs and treatments for COPD are constantly being refined,
and new ones are being developed. Just within the last few years, several
new medicines have been introduced that relieve spasm of bronchial tubes
or relieve inflammation of the mucous membrane. These are better than our
older medicines in that they may have either fewer side effects or longer duration of action, are in a more convenient form to take, may prevent spasm
(rather than treat it after it occurs), or may be more effective or less costly.

Although "new" does not mean "better" by any means (!) some of these "new" medicines may be "better" for you.

Recently, there has been some exciting research suggesting that retinoids (derivatives of vitamin A) is important in lung growth and that its use can restore lung function in some experimental models of emphysema. Although this has not yet been tried in human patients, a few experimental studies are under way in selected persons to determine whether this is a feasible form of treatment.

Another example of what lies ahead concerns drugs for better treatment of infection. As discussed earlier, infections are caused by different kinds of invaders—bacteria, fungi, and viruses. Antibiotics are effective in treating infections caused by bacteria. Unfortunately, they are less effective against fungi and viruses. No antibiotic can treat the flu and other virus infections. But research already has provided some drugs that can prevent (or treat) certain kinds of virus and fungus infections, and the future in this area looks bright.

Lung surgery for patients with COPD is another area of intense interest. In patients with advanced emphysema, lung volume reduction surgery has gotten a lot of attention in recent years. LVRS involves removing areas of overinflated lung tissue so that remaining parts of the lung can function better. However, there are many unanswered questions about LVRS that make it difficult to decide when or for whom it should be performed—questions such as: How long do the benefits last? What are the risks? What patterns or types of emphysema does LVRS work best for? LVRS is now under intense study in research projects that, hopefully, will provide answers to these key questions within a few years.

Lung transplantation is another new surgical option for patients with severe lung diseases like COPD. We are still learning about lung transplantation. Questions that need answers include: Who *needs* a lung transplant? *When* should it be done? Is one "new" lung enough (versus two)? How can we preserve a potential donor lung longer (now it must be used within a few hours after removal)? How can we prevent lung rejection? Questions, questions, questions! All seeking answers. Research is the key. But, in the meantime, a number of patients with severe chronic lung disease have received a lung transplant and the pace is accelerating.

Despite the many questions that remain, we clearly have made substantial gains. Some of the biggest gains have been are in *education of the public* about the factors that contribute to disease. Young children are being taught the hazards of smoking in the hope that they will never *begin* to smoke. Smokers are being aided in their efforts to quit. Many agencies are working toward cleaning up our air, another source of lung pollution.

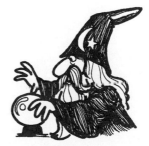

We are becoming aware of certain hazards to the lungs in the *workplace* (with asbestos being the most publicized) and are making progress in decreasing such hazards. Everywhere in our country, doctors and other medical personnel are becoming increasingly aware of chronic lung disease and are being trained in modern diagnosis and management. Pulmonary rehabilitation programs can help patients and families learn about lung disease and how to cope better and improve their function and quality of life. Research studies have demonstrated the benefits of such programs that are now more widely recognized as important in the care of patients with chronic lung disease.

The more that medical research discovers about chronic lung disease, the better doctors will be able to treat their patients. The *ultimate* goal is to learn enough so that chronic lung disease can be prevented. The key to achieving that goal is to assure that skilled researchers are trained and provided with the tools they need to continue the present pace of advancement.

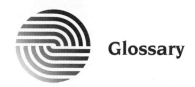 **Glossary**

accessory muscles — muscles used to supplement and assist the main muscles. Respiratory accessory muscle groups include the muscles of the upper chest, back, neck, and shoulders. They are usually at rest during quiet breathing and are used when extra breathing effort is needed.

acute — having a short course of illness or disease.

advance medical directive — these often include both a durable power of attorney for health care, which is a statement that outlines the medical treatments you would want, or names of the persons you would want to make health care decisions for you if you could no longer express your wishes, *and* a living will for end-of-life issues.

aerobic exercise — exercise that uses oxygen to fuel muscles.

aerosol — liquid or solid particles suspended in air.

aerosol medication — an aerosol of fine medication particles, delivered in airflow generated by a propellant or nebulizer (i.e., inhaled bronchodilators or steroids).

airways — tubes that carry air into and out of the lungs, called the trachea and bronchial tubes.

allergen — an internal or external substance to which a person is allergic.

allergy — abnormal reaction response to a stimulus, acquired by exposure to a particular allergen. Allergies are principally manifested in the skin, respiratory, and gastrointestinal tracts.

alpha 1 antitrypsin deficiency — a rare hereditary deficiency of alpha antitrypsin, a protective material in our lungs.

alveoli (plural), **alveolus** (singular) — air sacs in the lung, located at the ends of the smallest airways. The alveoli are where oxygen and carbon dioxide are exchanged in the lung. The alveoli are surrounded by capillary blood vessels, which bring blood to the lung to pick up oxygen and drop off carbon dioxide.

antibiotic — a drug that kills or inhibits the growth of microorganisms, such as bacteria. Antibiotics are effective in combating deep bacterial chest infections. It should be stressed that antibiotics do not prevent the common cold and will not stop a cold that has developed.

Arm-R-Size — unsupported, upper extremity endurance exercises.

arterial blood gas (ABG) — blood drawn from an artery, usually in your wrist, used to measure the levels of oxygen and carbon dioxide in the blood, used to assess how your lungs are working. Can be used to determine whether you would benefit from supplemental oxygen. The main function of the lung is to bring fresh oxygen to the body tissues and get rid of carbon dioxide. The arterial oxygen and carbon dioxide pressure levels are measured in millimeters of mercury. The percent of oxygen that is carried in your blood is also measured. The pH tells about the acid-base balance in your blood.

assertiveness — behaving in a boldly self-confident manner.

asthma — an obstructive lung disease that is characterized by airway narrowing, spasm, and inflammation. Wheezing is often heard as the air tries to move through constricted airways. In between asthma attacks, a person may have perfectly normal lung function. Once an attack starts, flow rate (speed at which air moves through the lung) will be reduced. Peak flow meters can be used to monitor your flow rate so you will be warned of any decrease in flow rates before you feel symptoms.

autogenic drainage — a bronchial hygiene, secretion-clearance technique that employs increasing lung volumes, breath holding, expiratory air flows, and coughing.

autonomic nervous system — the portion of the nervous system that regulates the activity of various organs, such as the heart, lungs, smooth muscles, and glands.

bacteria — infectious microorganisms that cause disease, such as bronchitis and pneumonia.

belly breathing — breathing techniques that use the muscles of the abdomen to aid respiration.

blood pressure — the force your blood is exerting on the walls of the blood vessels. Blood pressure is measured in millimeters of mercury and consists of two numbers (e.g., 120/80). The top number (or systolic pressure) reflects the highest pressure when your heart contracts; the bottom number (or diastolic pressure) reflects the pressure when the heart relaxes between beats.

Borg Scale — a scale to rate severity of symptoms. It is used commonly in pulmonary rehabilitation programs for rating perceived symptoms like breathlessness and muscle fatigue.

breathless — without breath; often used to describe feeling out of breath.

bronchi — tubes that carry the air into and out of the lungs. Bronchi branch into the right and left lungs. The main bronchi branch more than 20 times to form thousands of smaller bronchial tubes and bronchioles.

bronchial hygiene — treatment modalities that aid in the removal of irritants and secretions from the lungs.

bronchiectasis — structural distortion of the bronchial tubes caused by damage to the cartilage and muscle tissue. The damage is usually the result of a severe lower respiratory infection occurring early in life, during the development of the bronchial tubes.

bronchitis — inflammation of the bronchial tubes, characterized by coughing and production of mucus.

bronchodilator — a medication used to open or dilate the bronchial tubes.

bronchospasm — sudden contraction of the muscles surrounding the bronchi that results in narrowing of the airways.

bullae or **bleb** — large, abnormal air spaces in the lungs caused by the destruction of walls of neighboring alveoli. They are ineffective for oxygen–carbon dioxide exchange and can compress areas of otherwise functioning lung tissue.

capillaries — the smallest blood vessels. In the lungs capillaries form a network of semipermeable membranes, which allow for the interchange of oxygen and carbon dioxide.

carbon dioxide — gaseous metabolic waste product, exhaled by the lungs.

cardiopulmonary resuscitation (CPR) — a life-sustaining measure to temporarily reestablish heart and lung action, often used when the heart stops.

cardiovascular — pertaining to the heart and blood vessels.

central nervous system — the brain, spinal cord, and main nerve branches.

chest physiotherapy (CPT) — techniques used to aid clearance of mucus from the airways and lungs.

chronic — of long duration, prolonged, lingering.

cilia — minute hairlike structures on cell bodies, which beat rhythmically to move a mucus film over the surface. In the bronchial tubes, the cilia beat rhythmically upward to move mucus toward the mouth.

concentrator — medical device that takes in room air, filters out all but oxygen molecules (concentrating them) for delivery to patients.

congestive heart failure (CHF) — weakening of the heart, allowing buildup of fluid in the body.

cool-down exercises — exercises done gradually, more slowly, with less intensity to allow the body to cool down after a more vigorous exercise session.

COPD — chronic obstructive pulmonary disease; also called COAD (chronic obstructive airway disease) or COLD (chronic obstructive lung disease).

cor pulmonale — failure of the right side of the heart, usually caused by lung disease.

correct breathing technique (CBT) — pursed lips and belly breathing techniques used together.

corticosteroid — a hormone from adrenal gland, often used as an anti-inflammatory medication.

cystic fibrosis (CF) — a hereditary disease that often affects the lungs, in which there is widespread dysfunction of mucus-producing glands. Characterized by severe, chronic pulmonary disease with excess mucus produced in the respiratory tract.

desaturation — when saturation levels fall. Often used in reference to oxygen saturation.

diaphragm — the muscle and membrane partition that separates the chest (thorax) and abdomen. The major breathing muscle.

DME or **HME** — durable medical equipment or home medical equipment (supplier).

do not resuscitate (DNR) — a request or order not to use heroic measures to revive a person whose heart has stopped or who has stopped breathing.

dyspnea — a medical term used to describe someone else's difficulty breathing.

edema — swelling due to retention of abnormally large amounts of fluid in body tissues.

emphysema — a lung disease caused by overdistention, loss of elasticity, and/or rupture of the air sacs (alveoli) in the lungs.

endurance exercise — exercise that can be continued for a prolonged period of time.

epiglottis — a lidlike structure in the back of the throat that prevents food from entering the airways during swallowing.

exercise prescription — a prescription for an appropriate and safe amount of exercise.

exercise stress test — a medically monitored, maximum physical exercise test.

exercise target — the work rate in an exercise prescription.

exhale — to breathe out.

feedback — a means of returning information.

FEV1 — forced expiratory volume in 1 second, the maximal amount of air that can be exhaled forcefully in 1 second.

fibrosis — a condition that causes scarring.

flutter valve — medical device to aid in pulmonary secretion removal.

FVC — forced vital capacity, the total volume of air that can be forcefully exhaled after a maximal inhalation.

generic — nonproprietary, a product not protected by a patent or a trademark name.
genetic — inherited.
goblet cells — mucus-producing glands.

hemoglobin — the oxygen-carrying pigment in red blood cells.
holistic — emphasizing the importance of the whole and the interdependence of its parts.
hypoxemia — low level of oxygen in the blood.
hypoxia — low level of oxygen.

idiopathic — from an unknown cause.
inflammation — protective response characterized by pain, redness, heat, swelling, irritability, loss of function, and, if chronic, scarring.
inhale or **inspire** — to breathe in.
inspiratory muscles — muscles used to take in a breath.
intercostal muscles — muscles between the ribs.
intermittent pulse/demand oxygen delivery system — an oxygen delivery system that opens a valve to deliver a "pulse" quantity of oxygen, on inhalation "demand," and closes the valve during exhalation.
interstitial — within or between structural cell layers.
intimacy — close association, familiarity, or being intimate.
IPF — can be either Idiopathic Pulmonary Fibrosis, disease of fibrous scarring in the lungs of unknown cause, or Interstitial Pulmonary Fibrosis, fibrous scarring between the structural cell layers within the lung.

liquid oxygen — oxygen that has been cooled to its critical temperature (approximately –300°F), causing the molecules to get so close together that they form a liquid.
lung volume reduction surgery (LVRS) — surgery to remove areas of pulmonary emphysema, to allow more natural function of the surrounding, more normal lung tissue.

macrophage — free roving scavenger cells that can capture and digest contaminants within the lungs. Often called the clean-up crew or garbage collector cells.
meditation — an exercise in contemplation, a technique to attain a state of physical relaxation and psychological calm.
metabolism — the complex of physical and chemical processes involved in the maintenance of life.
metered dose inhaler, metered dose device (MDI, MDD, puffer) — an aerosol medication, inhalation delivery device, which measures and delivers a predetermined amount of medication per dose.
mucous membranes — special layer of delicate cells that line the upper and lower respiratory surfaces, such as nose, mouth, and bronchial tubes, as well as the digestive tract.
mucus — a sticky lubricating fluid that coats all mucous membranes.

nebulizer — a device to turn liquid medication into a fine mist or spray for inhalation.
nutrients — nourishing ingredients in food.

oximeter — a photoelectric device for determining oxygen saturation of the blood.
oxygen — a gaseous element essential in the respiration of plants and animals.
oxygen cannula — a small tube for the delivery of oxygen.
oxygen concentrator — a medical device for the separation, concentration, and delivery of oxygen from other components in atmospheric air.

oxygen conserving device — medical device reservoirs and demand delivery regulators to maximize oxygen delivery during inhalation, conserving oxygen supply during exhalation, and therefore extending use time of an oxygen delivery system.

oxygen cylinder — compressed oxygen gas container.

oxygen saturation — amount of oxygen attached to the hemoglobin, expressed as a percentage.

oxygen system — an oxygen container and means of delivery to a user.

peak flow (PF) — measurement of maximum velocity of exhaled airflow.

peak flow meter — a device for measuring peak flow.

PEP — positive expiratory pressure.

phlegm — mucus.

physiology — study of the physical parts and chemical functions of living organisms.

pleura — a thin membrane that lines the chest cavity and encases the lungs.

postural drainage (PD) — body positioning to use gravity to drain mucus from the lungs, also called bronchial drainage (BD).

processed foods — any food that has been processed beyond, or in any way has been altered from, its natural state.

pulmonary fibrosis — scarring in the lung.

pulmonary function testing — tests to measure how well the lungs work.

pulmonary hypertension — high blood pressure in the blood vessels in the lung.

pulmonary rehabilitation — a preventive health care program, provided by a team of health care professionals, including doctors, nurses, and respiratory care and exercise therapists, to help patients with lung diseases attain their maximum possible level of function and improve their quality of life.

pursed lips breathing (PLB) — exhaling with lips puckered to restrict and slow airflow.

respiration — the exchange of oxygen and carbon dioxide between the atmosphere and the cells of the body.

respiratory failure — when lungs cannot maintain an adequate balance of oxygen and carbon dioxide.

saline solution — salt water.

secretions — fluid exudates.

SOB — short of breath.

sodium — a chemical element contained in salts.

spacer — a medical device to put space between a metered dose inhaler and the mouth.

spirometry — a simple and brief pulmonary function/breathing test.

sputum — expectorated pulmonary secretions.

steroid — name generally applied to groups of naturally occurring hormones and fat-soluble compounds used to promote growth and repair body tissues.

strength — state, quality, or property of being strong; physical power.

strengthening exercises — exercises done repetitively to improve strength.

symptom — an abnormal sensation, often indicating disease.

thorax — the part of the body between the neck and the abdomen. The chest, including the diaphragm.

trachea — the cartilaginous and membranous tube descending from the larynx and branching into the right and left mainstem bronchial tubes. The windpipe.

tracheostomy — the surgical creation of an opening through the neck into the trachea.

transtracheal oxygen — oxygen delivery through the tracheal wall (windpipe) with the use of a very small catheter.

ventilator — a breathing machine to aid or control ventilation.

virus — one of a group of submicroscopic organisms, which can replicate only within living host cells and may cause disease.

visualization — a relaxation technique that uses the ability to mentally visualize images that can assist in reducing stress and promoting calm.

vital capacity — the amount of air that can be forcibly expelled from the lungs after a maximal inhalation.

warm-up exercise — exercise performed slowly to warm up the muscles of the body, increasing heart rate, breathing, and circulation, before a complete and more intense exercise session.

wheeze — the high-pitched sound made by air moving through narrowed air passages. A sign of bronchospasm or swelling in the airways, as in asthma.

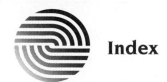

Index